Portraits
Catalogue II

William Harvey

Aged about 43, *c.* 1627, by an unknown artist (possibly by Joachim von Sandrart)

By courtesy of the Trustees of the National Portrait Gallery.
Portrait, formerly at Rolls Park, now the property of the National Portrait Gallery
(see footnote, Catalogue I, 1964, p. 214)

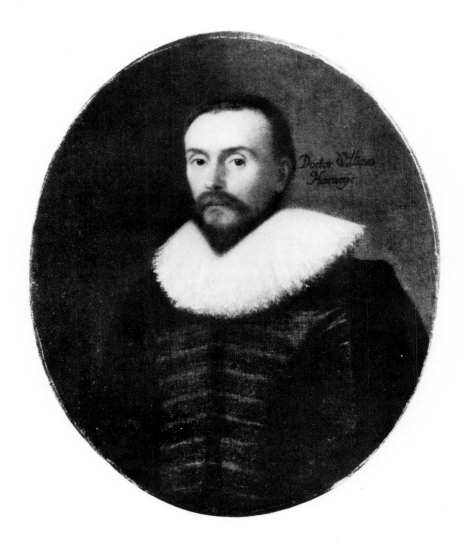

The Royal College
of Physicians of London

Portraits

Catalogue II

by
Gordon Wolstenholme F.R.C.P.
The Ciba Foundation

and

John F. Kerslake F.S.A.
National Portrait Gallery

With Essays by
Rudolf E.O. Ekkart and David Piper

1977

Elsevier • Excerpta Medica • North Holland

Amsterdam • Oxford • New York

ISBN Excerpta Medica 90 219 9291 4
ISBN Elsevier/North-Holland 0 444 15265 2

Published in 1977 by Elsevier/Excerpta Medica/North-Holland, P.O. Box 221, Amsterdam and Elsevier/North-Holland, 52 Vanderbilt Avenue, New York, N.Y. 10027.

Suggested publisher's entry for library catalogues: Elsevier/Excerpta Medica/North-Holland

Library of Congress Cataloging in Publication Data (Revised)

Wolstenholme, Gordon E   W   ed.
    The Royal College of Physicians of London.

Vol. 2 published by Elsevier/Excerpta Medica/North-
Holland, Amsterdam, and American Elsevier, New York.
    Includes bibliographies and index.
    CONTENTS: v. 1.   The portraits described by D. Piper.
--v 2.   The portraits described by J. F. Kerslake, with
essays by R. E. O. Ekkart and D. Piper.
    1. Physicians--Great Britain--Portraits--Catalogs.
2. Portraits, British--Catalogs.   3.   Portraits--England
--London--Catalogs.   4.   Royal College of Physicians of
London.   I.   Royal College of Physicians of London.
R489.A1W6   704.94′2′094107402142   64-1523

Printed in The Netherlands by Casparie-Alkmaar/IJsselstein.

Preface

In 1964 the Trustees of the Ciba Foundation produced a large illustrated catalogue of portraits in the collection of the Royal College of Physicians of London. The book was edited by myself, David Piper described the portraits, and the publishers were J. & A. Churchill Ltd. of London.

Since 1964 the College has acquired more than 60 additional portraits and a few which were not to be found earlier have now been traced. I have, therefore, undertaken to provide a supplementary volume, including biographical notes on the sitters, and this time with the portraits described by John Kerslake, Deputy Keeper of the National Portrait Gallery.

In this second volume, we are privileged to include an introductory article by Dr Rudolf E. O. Ekkart, Keeper of the Historical Museum of the University of Leiden, and also the 1974 Lloyd-Roberts Lecture given by Mr David Piper, now Director of the Ashmolean Museum, Oxford.

The first Catalogue was dedicated to 'The President and Fellows of the Royal College of Physicians of London'. This second Catalogue is fittingly dedicated to the present President, Sir Cyril Clarke, FRS, whose continued appreciation of the earlier work has inspired this further effort.

The production of Catalogue II would hardly have been possible without the scholarly and enthusiastic collaboration of Mr Leonard Payne, Hon. FRCP, during the closing months of his long and splendid service as Librarian to the College.

I am indebted to Megan Haddow for preparing perceptive preliminary notes on many of the sitters, from material in Munk's *Roll*, the *Dictionary of National Biography*, obituary notices in the press, and entries in *Who's Who* and the *Medical Directory*.

Gordon Wolstenholme

V

Editor's note

The portraits are in alphabetical order, by name or title of the sitter, as in Catalogue I.

Measurements of the portraits are given in inches; in the descriptions of paintings the height is given before the width, and the dimensions are those of the painted surface. The terms *left* and *right* always refer to the spectator's left and right, except where a specific indication is given that they refer to the sitter's left or right.

Where other portraits of persons represented in the College are known to exist, a note of them is generally given at the end of the entry, but no claim is made that these notes are exhaustive.

The following abbreviations are used in the text:

al. – refers to autograph letters in the College archives.

R.C.P. or College – refers to Royal College of Physicians of London.

N.P.G. – refers to National Portrait Gallery.

R.A. – refers to Royal Academy.

R.S.P.P. – refers to Royal Society of Portrait Painters.

Bibliography

Catalogue I, 1964 – *The Royal College of Physicians of London Portraits*, ed. by Gordon Wolstenholme, portraits described by David Piper, London, 1964.

Annals – refers to the manuscript *Annals*, or Minutes, of the College, in the keeping of the College.

Commentary – Royal College of Physicians of London, *College Commentary*.

Burgess, 1973 – R. BURGESS, *Portraits of Doctors and Scientists in the Wellcome Institute for the History of Medicine*, London, 1973.

Driver, 1952 – A. H. DRIVER, *Catalogue of Engraved Portraits in the Royal College of Physicians of London*, London, 1952.

Forrer	L. S. Forrer, *Biographical Dictionary of Medallists*, London, 1904–30. 6 vols. and 2 supplements.
Freeman	S. E. Freeman, *Medals Relating to Medicine . . . in the Numismatic Collection of the Johns Hopkins University, a Catalogue*, Baltimore, Md. 1964.
Hawkins	E. Hawkins and others, *Medallic Illustrations of the History of Great Britain and Ireland*, London, 1885. 2 vols.
LeFanu	W. R. LeFanu, *A Catalogue of the Portraits and Other Paintings, Drawings and Sculpture in the Royal College of Surgeons of England*, Edinburgh, 1960.
List	– *List of the Fellows and Members of the Royal College of Physicians of London*, London, 1973.
O'Donoghue	– F. O'Donoghue, *Catalogue of Engraved British Portraits Preserved in the Department of Prints and Drawings in the British Museum*, London, 1908–25, 6 vols.
Storer	– H. R. Storer, *Medicina in Nummis; a descriptive list of the Coins, Medals, Jetons relating to Medicine*, ed. M. Storer, Boston, 1931.

Acknowledgments

It is a pleasure to acknowledge the cooperation of the officers of the Royal College of Physicians, especially Dr. C. E. Newman, Mr. L. M. Payne and Miss D. P. Quayle. In the National Museums several colleagues mentioned in the text lent their expertise in fields far from mine. Mr. J. V. Murrell kindly examined the miniatures and Mr. M. Powell-Jones, the coins. In all these instances, the mistakes are mine, the merit theirs.

John Kerslake   VII

Contents

Dedicated by the Editor and his colleagues to

Sir Cyril Clarke, **K.B.E., M.D., F.R.S.**

President of the Royal College of Physicians 1972–1977

Collections of portraits in Western Europe

Rudolf E. O. Ekkart

A visitor to the building of the Royal College of Physicians of London in Regent's Park (Figs. 1 and 11) runs no risk of being bored during a stroll through the halls, auditoriums and rooms, since he will find everywhere examples of a portrait collection, consisting of hundreds of portraits, with the names of famous English portrait artists such as Lely, Kneller, Reynolds, Zoffany and Lawrence. On further inspection, however, he will discover that from an artistic viewpoint a great number of the portraits are of moderate or even mediocre quality, and after passing through all the rooms of the building he will note that many artists, who have played an essential part in English portrait art, are missing from the collection. But the visitor who inspects the collection solely from the viewpoint of art history has chosen an erroneous approach. It is not the quality of the paintings and sculpture that is representative, nor the names of the artists who executed them. A collection such as the one in the Royal College of Physicians has been brought together to preserve in an appropriate manner for posterity the features of as large a number of persons as possible who during their lifetime kept close ties with the College or who earned in other ways the interest or admiration of English doctors. Portrait galleries like this one have the remarkable characteristic that they can contain important works of art, more or less by chance, next to works of little artistic significance. In this regard the collection of the Royal College of Physicians hardly distinguishes itself from most of the portrait galleries of universities and learned societies and it is therefore justifiable to view the birth and growth of this collection in the context of the history of similar galleries. For this we have to go back several stages in European history.

Collecting portraits is probably almost as old as portrait art itself. However, we can trace a more or less continuous development from the Middle Ages. From the 13th century, in various places, portrait collections were made that we can best describe as 'galleries of rulers'; they were no doubt inspired by the series of busts of Roman emperors and were made up of a series of likenesses of all successive rulers of a certain area. In this way the succession of monarchs could be shown visually and the monarch of the moment was placed in a centuries long tradition, which

1

clearly underlined the legality of his own authority.[1] We know that there were such series in France, Germany and Italy. For instance, in Rome and Pisa, the successive Popes – who were then not only spiritual but also worldly rulers – were portrayed.[2] In the following centuries we find examples of this sort of gallery in practically all European countries, including England, where according to a legend transmitted by Dugdale a portrait series of English kings was present as a mural in the dining-hall of the abbot of the monastery of St. Peter at Gloucester in the first quarter of the 14th century.[3] The earliest examples in England to remain preserved, however, only date from the end of the 15th century. They are a few busts and half figures in oil on panels in Windsor Castle[4] and three life-sized full-length figures, also oils on panel, from Baston Manor in Kent,[5] all of them representing English kings. In other countries one can find more complete series, such as, for example, in Holland, where in the City Hall of Haarlem a series of the counts of Holland is preserved. These paintings were made shortly after 1500 and were copied from murals in a cloister in Haarlem dating from approximately 1420.[6]

Obviously, in such portraits one cannot have too high expectations regarding the likeness of those depicted; the portraits of the early monarchs were first made centuries after their death and can be regarded as totally fictitious portraits. In many of the series made in England and elsewhere in the 16th century we see that the fantasy portraits of older generations are supplemented with copies of more or less trust-worthy pictures of 15th and 16th century monarchs.[7]

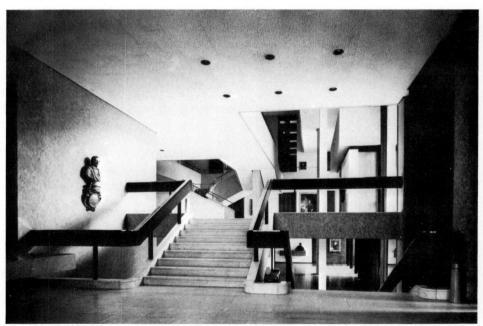

2   *Fig. 1.* Main Hall, St. Andrew's Place

Although by the 16th century such series had lost practically all of their function as visual proof of the rights of the ruling monarch, it is in this period that they experienced an hitherto unknown popularity, probably in many cases mainly as a symbol of a bond with the ruling dynasty, sometimes as an expression of purely historical interest. At any rate, in that century countless copies in painted and printed form found their way into official buildings and into the homes of well-to-do individuals. The example was followed at lower levels of society, the lesser nobility and rich citizens establishing family galleries in which pictures of the successive generations and sometimes also of other relations were brought together.[8]

An essential characteristic of this sort of portrait gallery is the almost total lack of choice: the historical succession had to be respected, so that, for example, deposed rulers had to be included, and also the presence of a portrait of a black sheep in the family whenever he formed an indispensable link in the lineage.

There was much more freedom of choice in variants of a completely other type of portrait gallery, best described by the Italian term *ritratti di uomini famosi*, portraits of famous men. This genre of portrait series also goes back to examples from Roman times. The purpose at that time was to bring together a number of portraits of persons who in some way could be held as examples to a later generation. Sometimes, especially in Germanic speaking areas, the choice was not free but portrayed the traditional three pagan, three Jewish and three Christian heroes (The Nine Worthies)[9], also sometimes personally selected figures, for example from persons described in Petrarch's '*De viris illustribus*'.[10] These were usually small series of paintings, although occasionally somewhat larger, such as, for example, the series of 28 portraits in the *studiolo* of Federigo da Montefeltro in Urbino, executed by Justus of Gent and Pedro Berruguete in approximately 1475–1480.[11] In the history of this sort of gallery of famous men a highlight was the decoration of the *Sala theatri* in the Orsini Palace at Monte Giordano in Rome, commissioned by Cardinal Giordano Orsini and executed by Masolino and Uccello, about 1430. In its entirety it contained not less than 300 full-length portraits of *uomini famosi*, unfortunately lost later in the 15th century by acts of war.[12]

In spite of their differences, the mediaeval and early-Renaissance portrait galleries discussed up till now had one important common similarity: none of them were collections obtained by gathering individual pieces, but rather the result of a single commission to one or more artists, while additions were made later on in order to keep the gallery up-to-date. The creation of true collections of this kind is a phenomenon that became established only in the 16th century. Its prototype was to be found in the activities of Paolo Giovio, whose example exercised great influence throughout most of Europe.

Paolo Giovio (1483–1552), Bishop of Nocera dei Pagani, began to collect portraits of famous men in 1521, when he was still living in Rome. He preferred small paintings approximately 12 inches in height and demanded close resemblance in the portraits. In well over 30 years Giovio brought together not less than 360 pictures, divided into four sections that he himself devised, namely, deceased poets and scholars, living poets and scholars, artists, and statesmen and soldiers.[13] Even during Giovio's lifetime his collection gained international fame, and several persons had copies made of his paintings so that they could establish their own galleries of famous men.[14] Of even greater significance than these painted copies were the prints made after portraits from his collection. The first edition of his biographies of famous men, which appeared shortly before Giovio's death, was illuminated with only a few woodcuts, but in the years 1575–1577 an edition was published with approximately 200 woodcuts of drawings that the German artist Tobias Stimmer had made in 1570–1571 of paintings from Giovio's collection.[15] Apparently a good market developed at that time for similar publications illustrated with portraits, for example the appearance in 1567 and 1572 of books with copper engravings of portraits of scholars by Philips Galle from Antwerp.[16] The prints of Galle and Stimmer enjoyed wide distribution and contributed greatly to the design of the scholar portrait. Many publications of this sort appeared in the last quarter of the 16th century and in the following centuries, while these prints were often used as the basis for painted portraits of scholars. In many places in Europe collections were assembled which comprised portraits of famous persons, collections that frequently were adapted to local circumstances and often were mixed with family portraits and royalty of the particular country. In this manner, older portrait series could be incorporated into this new genre; one's own forefathers might be displayed alongside the great of the world.[17] One of the most important English examples of such a portrait collection from the last quarter of the 16th century is that of John, Lord Lumley of Lumley Castle.[18]

What especially distinguished the collection of Giovio and the collections that arose under his influence from the galleries of *uomini famosi* of the Middle Ages and early Renaissance is the escape from limited representation of persons out of the past, so that famous persons out of both distant and recent past, as well as contemporaries, could be shown next to each other. In this respect Giovio was also of great significance for the formation of those portrait galleries that shortly before and after 1600 began to take shape at universities and learned societies. The oldest known examples of these are to be found in Germany, the Netherlands and England. Unfortunately, only rarely can one establish precisely when such collections began. It is quite possible that this happened in Leipzig soon after the middle of the 16th century, and in other German universities such as Jena and Tübingen just a few decades later.[19] A memorandum from 1597 is particularly informative. Written by the Librarian of the still young University of Leiden, he proposed to collect copper engravings of all important scholars together with painted portraits of the founder of the university, of the most important professors of Leiden and of the most famous Dutch writers from the fairly distant and recent past.[20]

Nothing much came of the scheme to collect engravings, but the collection of oil paintings, although initially modest in size, met approximately the demands set in

1597.[21] This collection in Leiden was not so similar to the German collections of the time which concentrated mainly on the portraits of local professors, as to the English collections which were being formed at the same time. There too we see a combination in the first place of founders and benefactors, secondly of professors of the institute itself and thirdly of famous scholars and writers from elsewhere. We know with certainty that after the eighties of the 16th century portraits of founders and benefactors and university functionaries were to be found in the various colleges of Oxford and Cambridge. The addition of other portraits followed rapidly.[22] The best example of such a heterogenous collection is that in the Bodleian Library in Oxford, where shortly after its opening in 1602, the first work, a marble bust of the founder Sir Thomas Bodley, was installed and where in the following centuries there grew a very extensive collection of portraits of persons not necessarily related to Oxford.[23] A particular example is the frieze painted between 1616 and 1620 above the bookcases, with a total of 200 portraits of writers from all periods.[24]

In regard to heterogeneity, the statute of April 5, 1596, of the Royal College of Physicians of London comes as no surprise. It was then determined that if any member or any noble person from outside the college wished to donate his portrait or coat of arms as an everlasting remembrance, he was free to do so provided that the portrait or coat of arms concerned were made at his own expense or that of his friends, and that a sum of 10 pounds were paid to the College. However, a President of the College who had served for not less than three years was allowed to hang his portrait or coat of arms without having to pay a similar amount.[25] The stipulation that one had to deposit money in order to have the right to hang a portrait or coat of arms constitutes a remarkable and rare element. The inference is that in this way the funds of the College were to profit by it. The rest of the text of the statute is in accordance with what could be expected in those times: the first intention was to obtain portraits of Fellows of the Royal College, but if others (implying most likely visiting foreign doctors) wished to donate a portrait, that was also very welcome. Especially interesting is the fact that Presidents of the College were encouraged to donate a portrait or coat of arms by exempting them from paying a contribution to the treasury. This is in line with the characteristics of other collections, where special attention was paid to the gathering of a series of portraits of the highest authorities, such as the Chancellors of the universities or, as in the Bodleian, the foremost writers. In German universities this phenomenon was carried much further, in some places almost exclusively including rectors of the university and deans of the faculty, resembling the old galleries of rulers.

Unfortunately, it is impossible to determine with certainty how much success the London statute of 1596 has had. It is certain that in the financial administration of the College no traces have been found that indicate payment of 10 pounds as levy for the hanging of portraits or coats of arms. We do know that in 1662 a number of portraits was present in the building in Amen Corner, where the Royal College of Physicians was established since 1614 – after having made use of the home of the first President, Thomas Linacre; since the creation of the College in 1518.[26] In 1662 John Evelyn noted down that he was taken through the building by the librarian and that he had seen a statue of Dr. William Harvey and painted portraits of Dr. William Gilbert, Sir William Paddy and others. The statue of Harvey had been made in 1652 by order of the College, and was followed in 1656 by the commission of a marble bust of Dr. Simeon Foxe. All these portraits, however, were lost in the Great Fire of 1666, when the building in Amen Corner was destroyed. In addition to a number of books and annals, only two paintings could then be saved, a portrait of Harvey and one of Foxe of whom there had been a painting as well as a sculpture. The portrait of Foxe was lost later on, so that the large painted portrait of Harvey which presently adorns the walls of the College forms the only reminder of the Collection before 1666.

After the Great Fire it was years before money could be found for the construction of a new building for the College. Eventually, between 1674–1679, a newly built establishment in Warwick Lane could be taken into use. The portrait of Harvey received a place of honour in the Long Room where the doctors gathered every three months. The further decoration of the exterior and interior of the building could then be tackled. Eighty pounds were spent for two facade statues (Fig. 2, 3) executed by the sculptor 'Colein', likenesses of King Charles II and of Sir John Cutler, the man who had made the construction of the new building financially possible.[27] Bij 1680, a marble bust of the late Baldwin Hamey junior, a Fellow of the College, had been purchased as a decoration for the interior, while in this period the first donations of portraits began to arrive.

The first benefactor was Sir Edmund King, who offered in 1682 a painted portrait of the former President Sir John Micklethwaite, who had died earlier that year. A few years later Sir Theodore Colladon followed by donating a portrait of Sir Theodore de Mayerne, the personal physician of King Charles I, while William Sydenham in 1691 gave a portrait of his illustrious father Thomas Sydenham. The Royal College of Physicians was very interested in expanding its collection; this appears from the fact that in the same year it commissioned a copy of a portrait of Henry Pierrepont, 1st Marquis of Dorchester, who had died 11 years earlier, and who had donated to the College after the Great Fire his own valuable library, as compensation for the loss. There was an interval of several years before the collection was further enlarged, but around the turn of the century a steady influx of paintings started. The College received a painted portrait of Baldwin Hamey junior, and portraits of the Presidents Daniel Whistler and Sir Thomas Millington, of the illustrious Sir Thomas Browne, and of Edmund Boulter, the nephew and executor of the Sir John Cutler mentioned earlier. This last portrait was probably given by Boulter himself and already hung in the College when he was still alive.

Sir Charles Goodall donated in 1706 two paintings that could not be omitted from such a collection, namely a portrait of King Henry VIII, the founder of the College, and of his adviser Cardinal Thomas Wolsey, whose influence on the king allegedly

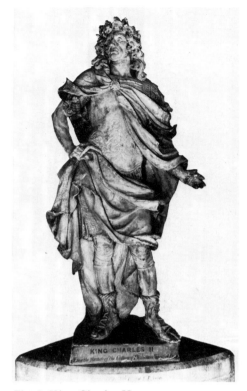

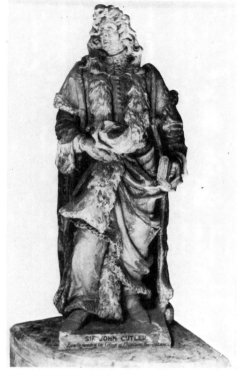

Fig. 2. King Charles II   *Fig. 3.* Sir John Cutler

made the foundation possible. Both paintings are quite mediocre copies of paintings elsewhere, but quality was not demanded of works in a collection such as this one.

Thanks to a description of the College that appeared in 1708,[28] we know where the majority of the above-mentioned works were located in the building in Warwick Lane (Fig. 4). In the Long Room were to be found the marble bust of Hamey and the three-quarter length oil portraits of Mayerne and Harvey, in the Censors' Room the whole-length portrait of Millington, the three-quarter length portraits of Hamey and Micklethwaite and the head and shoulders portraits of Whistler and Boulter. Whether the portraits which are not mentioned in the description also hung in these rooms, or whether they were given a place elsewhere, is not clear. Supposedly a painting such as that of Pierrepont, who had donated part of the book collection, hung in the library, as happened in many other learned societies. In any case, a few decades later the Physicians decorated their library also in this manner, for in 1729 it was decided to commission especially for the library a replica of a portrait of Dr. Richard Hale (Fig. 5), who had willed to the College a sum of 450 pounds.

In the course of the 18th century the portrait collection of the Royal College of   7

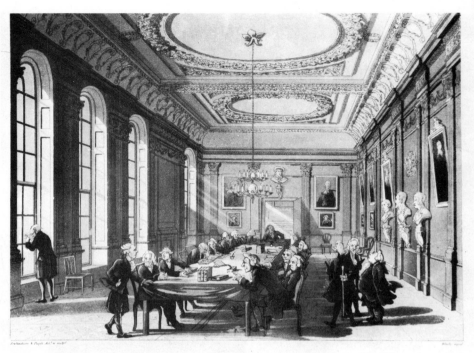

THE COLLEGE OF PHYSICIANS.

Fig. 4. Long Room, Warwick Lane

Physicians was enlarged regularly by donations, so that by the end of the century there were more than 35 paintings and sculptures, a number that is tiny compared to the much more extensive collections brought together in the universities and in particular in Oxford. This difference in quantity was a result not only of the fact that in universities portraits of all sorts of writers, scholars, monarchs, politicians and artists found a place, whilst the College had only portraits of doctors and other persons closely connected with its history; it was also due to the fact that in the universities there was a much stronger tradition of donating portraits resulting in regular donations of works and sometimes even entire collections. The history of the College in London does not contain a donor such as Humphrey Bartholomew, who donated eight portraits of English doctors to the University of Oxford in 1735. Some of these portraits incidentally, were copies of paintings that belonged already to the collection of the College of Physicians.[29]

Although the London collection was of modest size, its history in the 18th century is of considerable interest, particularly because in that century a number of people had their portraits painted especially for the benefit of the College.

8   We have already referred to the various pictures of former Presidents which hung

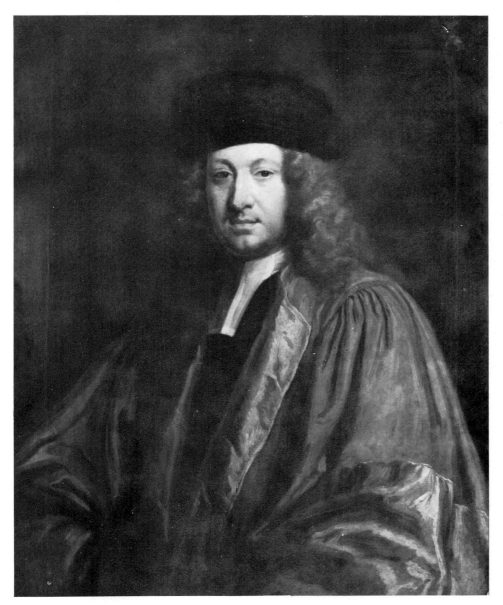

Fig. 5. Dr. Richard Hale

in the College building. One of these pictures, that of Millington, who died in 1704, came into the collection soon after his death. A few years later, in 1713, the widow of Charles Goodall, one of his successors, donated a portrait of her recently deceased husband, a painting which incidentally had been made long before Goodall

9

had assumed the presidency. No portraits of Goodall's immediate successors, Dawes and Bateman, were included in the collection, but Sir Hans Sloane, who wielded the presidential hammer for no less than 16 years from 1719 to 1735, opened a new tradition. Sloane appears to have donated during his presidency a three-quarter length picture of himself, which was the first time that a picture of a president still living came into the collection. It is no surprise that it was Sloane who initiated this new idea: on the one hand, as an inveterate collector he probably had more of an eye for the formation of a collection such as that in the Royal College than his co-fellows; on the other hand, his vanity probably also stimulated him to take this step. Moreover, the College of Physicians was not the only institution that he considered worthy enough to display his features to contemporaries and posterity, for he also donated portraits of himself to the Royal Society (of which he was President also) and to the Bodleian Library in Oxford.[30] Sloane's example was followed by his two immediate successors. Although there are no data to be found in the archives concerning the origin of his portrait, it seems likely that Thomas Pellett, President from 1735 to 1739, commissioned Michael Dahl to paint his portrait – dated 1737 – especially for the College and donated it directly after its completion. This is suggested by the fact that Pellett wears the President's gown in this painting, the earliest depiction of this official costume, which apparently was introduced by Pellett or perhaps by Sloane.[31] The same President's gown is to be seen in the portrait of Pellett's successor, Henry Plumptre, President from 1740 to 1745, who donated the portrait himself in 1744. Unfortunately, Plumptre's successors broke this tradition of presidential state portraits. It was twenty years later when the particularly vain Sir William Browne, after a turbulent presidency of two years (1765–1766), once again took up and even strengthened the neglected tradition: while his predecessors had had themselves depicted in three-quarter length, Browne chose, in spite or because of his small stature, a whole-length portrait in which he was depicted in the President's gown, with various other symbols: the Statutes, the President's Mace and the Caduceus (Fig. 6). Thus he obtained a state portrait of himself in the true meaning of the word. In 1767 he donated this picture, painted by Thomas Hudson, to the College.

After Browne the 'President's gallery' was not continued in the same stately manner. Two of the most important Presidents of the late 18th century, William Pitcairn and Sir George Baker, had themselves painted in the President's gown, even if only in half-length portraits, but they did not offer their pictures to the College. Only in the 19th century did their heirs hand over these portraits.

Of the 18th century acquisitions, we have discussed here almost exclusively the portraits of the Presidents of the College. Most of the other newly acquired pieces were pictures of doctors who had been dead for 50 years or more at the time their portraits were presented. An exception to this is made by two portraits, a painting and a marble bust, of Richard Mead, who died in 1754. Both portraits were donated just a few years after his death.

10

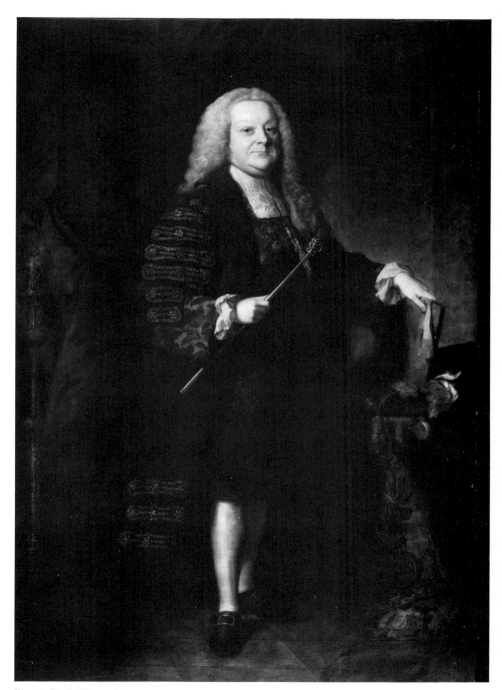

Fig. 6. Sir William Browne

If we look at the nucleus of the portrait collection of the Royal College of Physicians, obtained before 1800, from a viewpoint of art history, we must state that the average quality is not high, even though a small number of good to very good portraits can be indicated.

Of the few sculptures, the portrait bust of Hamey by Edward Pierce and that of Mead by Louis François Roubiliac deserve mention as good examples of sculpture of the second half of the 17th and the middle of the 18th centuries respectively.

Among the paintings we find numerous copies, which also vary greatly in quality among themselves, and a large group of originals of very meagre quality. The famous portrait of Harvey, the only remnant of the collection from before the Great Fire, must be included in the last group. Among the names of painters, those of Sir Peter Lely and Sir Godfrey Kneller are the best known. Lely's portrait of Edmund King cannot be included among his best works, while Kneller's picture of Garth is in fact a very good studio replica of the painting he made for the well-known portrait series of the Kit-cat Club.[32] Much more interesting are a few paintings by artists with somewhat lesser reputations, who in their works in the Royal College revealed their best, such as, for example, Jonathan Richardson, whose particularly fine portrait of Hale (present in two specimens almost equal in value) makes clear that this painter may be included among the best English portraitists of the first half of the 18th century. Richardson's son-in-law Thomas Hudson is also excellently represented in the College: his portrait of William Browne (Fig. 6) can be considered as a culminating-point in his artistic accomplishment. Edmund Lilley, a lesser known painter, active around 1700, excels here with a beautiful portrait of Edward Tyson, while the better known artists Michael Dahl, Thomas Murray and Mary Beale are represented with typical examples of their capabilities. Amongst the anonymous works the impressive picture of Sir Theodore de Mayerne deserves to be mentioned; it is a fine product of English portrait art from the middle of the 17th century. Moreover, a pleasant circumstance in collections such as the one in the Royal College of Physicians is the presence of a few signed or documented works of extremely rare masters, works that deserve attention not so much because of their outstanding quality, but because they have an important documentary value for the art historian. In this category may be counted Boulter's portrait by Morland and Hamey's portrait by Snelling.

Although the collection has increased enormously, in the 19th and 20th century the general character of its significance for art history remains unchanged. What has also remained is its iconographic character: it was and still is a collection of pictures chiefly of Fellows of the Royal College (among whom mainly many Presidents), of a few Licentiates and of a small number of other persons who were worthy of the doctors' admiration. Among the sitters one finds many of the most famous and most illustrious Fellows, on the one hand because their portraits were commissioned often at the expense of the College or individual members; on the other hand, probably because in these instances more pressure was placed on the heirs to donate a picture. Sometimes there appears, as we saw in the 18th century, a certain regularity in the acquisition of portraits of Presidents, but any such regularity was always soon interrupted, so that never could a reasonably complete 'President's gallery' develop. Looking through the catalogue of the College, we notice that many Fellows who were in no way outstanding, are also represented in the collection.

The collection has remained predominantly one of paintings. There are portrait busts in marble and bronze, but numerically they fall into a subordinate position, as opposed to some other collections such as that of the Royal College of Surgeons of England, founded in 1800, where a proportionately larger number of sculptures was acquired through commissions from the College or through donations.[33] The Physicians seem to have had in general a preference for paintings. A short review of the enlargement of the collection in the 19th and 20th centuries can illustrate this further.

The years between 1767 and 1824 were gloomy years for the expansion of the collection: as far as we know only one portrait was acquired in that period, and a bad purchase at that.[34] It is probable that the scant interest in those years was partly due to a lack of space in the building in Warwick Lane. The construction in 1825 of a new and more spacious establishment in Pall Mall East (Figs. 7 and 8) was the stimulus for new commissions and donations, amongst which also were several sculptures. The Fellows donated a bust of the President then in office, Sir Henry Halford, whose efforts to an important extent had made it possible to move into the

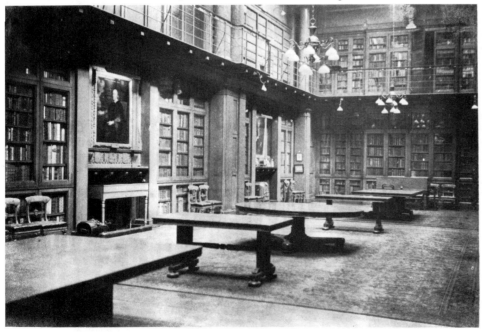

Fig. 7. Large Library, Pall Mall East

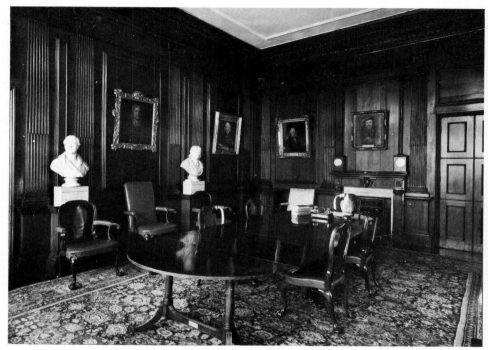

Fig. 8. Censors' Room, Pall Mall East (By permission of Country Life)

new building. At the opening ceremony King George IV presented a marble bust of himself, while the College commissioned the execution of a similar bust of Matthew Baillie, who had died in 1823. Private individuals donated a few paintings including the portrait of the former President Sir George Baker by Ozias Humphrey, and John Zoffany's portrait of William Hunter lecturing as Professor of Anatomy in the Royal Academy of Arts.

An interest in the collection of portraits was now definitely aroused and after 1825 a regular expansion can be noted. Amongst the works entering the collection before the middle of the century there are a few of special significance, namely the portraits of William Pitcairn by Sir Joshua Reynolds, of Sir Richard Jebb by John Zoffany, of David Pitcairn by John Hoppner, and of Matthew Baillie by Sir Thomas Lawrence. These paintings and those already present were almost without exception life-sized portraits at least 30 inches high. Apparently smaller paintings were not considered appropriate to keep alive the memory of a person. A clear example of this is the origin of the portrait of Pelham Warren who died in 1835. Shortly before his death Warren posed for the painter John Linnell, a specialist in small, lively portraits. His excellent portrait of Warren was only 15 by 11¾ inches large. Warren's widow decided to commission Linnell to make a life-sized (50 by 39¾) replica which she donated to the College in 1837. As far as its size was concerned this copy fitted

14

better into the collection, but a comparison with the original portrait, which luckily could be bought for the College at an auction in 1949, teaches us what a loss the blow-up to a larger size meant (Figs. 9 and 10). The pursuit of a certain uniformity in a portrait gallery sometimes involves an artistic loss, as in apparent in this case.

The expansion of the collection continued steadily in the second half of the 19th century. In this period over 70 pieces were acquired amongst which were a number of important additions to the material from the 17th and 18th century already present. It should be noted that the College, which up till then had only acted as a recipient of donations or as a sponsor of new portraits, now also acted as a purchaser of older paintings. In 1864 it bought the portrait believed to be of John Arbuthnot, now known to be of the 1st Earl of Mansfield – painted around 1738 by J. Vanloo – and in 1874 it bought the portrait – ascribed to Robert Streater – of Sir Francis Prujean, who was President of the College from 1650 to 1653. These purchases were the beginning of an active policy of collecting that in the 20th century was to bring many works within the walls of the buildings in Pall Mall East and St. Andrew's Place. In the 19th century the majority of the acquisitions were still donations. Among the contributors special mention should be made of Dr. Henry Monro, himself a Fellow of the College; in 1857 he donated four portraits of his father, grandfather, great-grandfather and great-great-grandfather, all Fellows of the Royal College, and in 1870 he added a self-portrait, so that a unique series of five consecutive generations was created.

As the collection grew during the 19th century, portraits were acquired of most of the Presidents: if we include pictures that were donated in the beginning of this century, all of the Presidents to have held office between 1813 and 1899 except one are represented, the majority depicted in the President's gown, and therefore probably specially portrayed for the College.[35] For no other period is there so complete a series of portraits of Presidents. Other acquisitions included portraits of more and of less well-known Fellows; the number of Fellows of whom there are portraits, sometimes painted posthumously, sometimes drawn from life, is much greater than in previous periods, but is relatively small when we realize that the number of Fellows of the College greatly increased during the 19th century.[36]

From the viewpoint of the history of art, the 19th century is well represented. The flowering of English portrait art ended with the death of Lawrence in 1830, but after that time there were still many masters who can be regarded as good representatives of English art, such as Frederick Richard Say, George Richmond, George Frederic Watts and Sir John Everett Millais. The latter was particularly valued in his time, as can be concluded from the insurance the Royal College of Physicians placed at that time on his portrait of Sir Richard Quain. In 1903 the building in Pall Mall East with its entire inventory was insured for the sum of £41,000, but since no individual piece was covered for more than £500, two paintings were insured separately for a total of £3,500, namely the portrait of Richard Warren, considered at that time to be an authentic Gainsborough (currently considered to

15

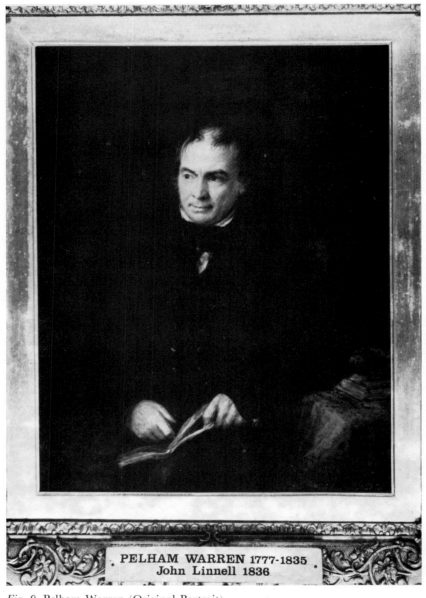

PELHAM WARREN 1777-1835
John Linnell 1836

16   *Fig. 9.* Pelham Warren (Original Portrait)

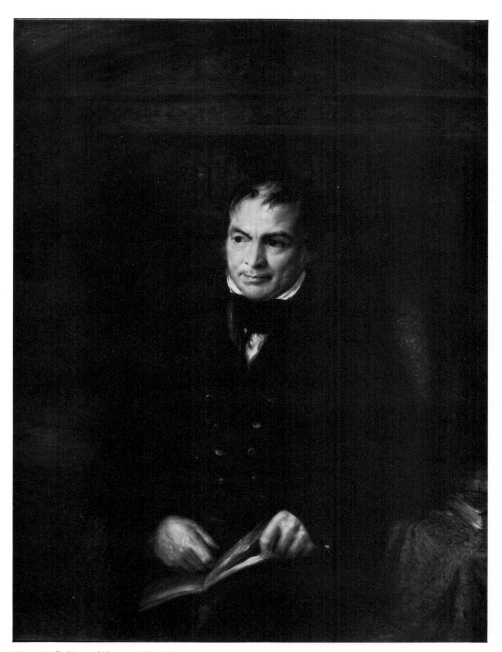

Fig. 10. Pelham Warren (Replica)

be a copy), and the painting by Millais.[37] The present evaluation is rather different, although the painting belongs to the best works of that period in the collection.

In 1875 statues were made to decorate the exterior of the building in Pall Mall. In the niches above the doors three statues of Linacre, Harvey and Sydenham were placed, made by Henry Weekes for a sum of more than 424 pounds. The statues remained in their places until the College moved in 1963, after which they came into the hands of private individuals who restored the badly damaged statues and placed them in their gardens.[38]

Mainly through the active buying policy of the Royal College rapid growth of the portrait collection continued in the 20th century. During both World Wars and the depression this growth was small, but in all other periods at least one or two works were added yearly, so that between 1900 and 1975 a total of 125 paintings, statues and drawings was obtained. In addition, we have the creation of collections of prints and photographs. In 1891 the print collection was founded with a legacy from Dr. James Butterworth, consisting of portraits of Fellows of the College and of other doctors. In 1934 Dr. Arnold Chaplin's donation represented a considerable enlargement. Through these and other additions the number of prints has grown to more than 4500.[39] A collection of photographs was created in order to establish a visual record of the rapidly growing number of Fellows.

A number of very important paintings from the 17th and 18th century have been acquired, including portraits of Sir Charles Scarburgh, John Allen and Edward Archer, but especially a large number of works from the 19th and 20th century among which are portraits of many important figures, including several Presidents. The fact that the collection is spread over a large number of hallways, halls and rooms in the building in St. Andrew's Place, occupied in 1964, means that the diversity of materials and sizes is not disturbing (Fig. 11).

During its existence of more than four and a half centuries the Royal College of Physicians has assembled a collection of painted, sculptured and drawn portraits of approximately 270 works. It is striking that from the first 150 years of its history only one portrait has been preserved; from the following 150 years a few dozen, and that more than 80% of the collection was acquired since 1825. In addition to the portraits, the collection contains a few other paintings such as a picture of the old building of the College in Pall Mall East, a painting attributed to George Dawe that carries the name 'The Maniac', and an interesting 17th century painting 'A Dwarf', that is very close to the work of the Flemish painter Jacob van Oost (Fig. 12).

Looking at the collection of the Royal College in its entirety, it is striking that very few of the portraits indicate the profession of the person portrayed, which is rather strange for a collection that was brought together mainly to represent one profession. There are, of course, a number of portraits, as we have mentioned, in which Presidents of the College had themselves depicted in their official robes. In a few dozen paintings those portrayed are characterized as scholars by the

18

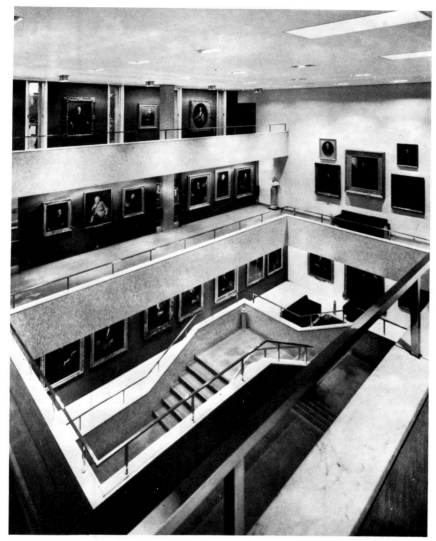

Fig. 11. Galleries, St. Andrew's Place

addition of one or more books, but only in a few works is there an indication that we are viewing a portrait of a medical man. Hamey, King and Freind had themselves depicted with a bust of Hippocrates, and in a few 19th and early 20th century portraits instruments indicate the activities of those portrayed; Richard Mead obviously did not wish to leave anything to chance in his portrait by an unknown artist from around 1740, and had himself portrayed with Minerva, a plaque with the head of Harvey and with a few medical books that have clearly legible names

19

on the back. Portraits of this kind, however, form a small minority, whereas in the vast majority of the portraits one cannot detect the profession of the person portrayed.

In no other country of the world has so much attention been directed to the collecting of portraits as in England, and in no other country can one find in so many

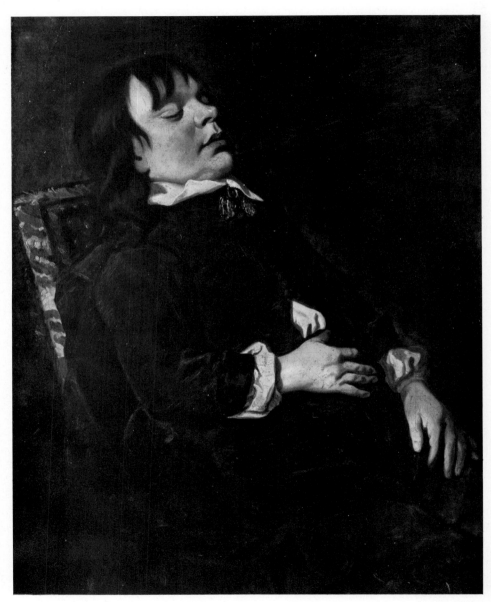

Fig. 12. The Dwarf

institutions of a social and cultural nature, collections of portraits which picture the history of the organization. These collections vary in size from a few objects to several thousands, and also show marked differences in regard to value. Unfortunately up till today only a part of them has been thoroughly studied, and there are few that are generally known through the publication of a printed catalogue. Therefore, it is difficult to place the significance of a certain collection in the total picture, and every remark made about it is somewhat premature. However, the collection of the Royal College of Physicians of London provides an important example, since in this portrait collection the history of this very old learned society is well reflected, whilst few other organizations have been able to give such a clear picture of their own past. The historical function of the portrait gallery of the College is strengthened by the unquestioned artistic qualities and the value for the history of art of a number of works, so that the conclusion is justified that the portrait collection of the Royal College of Physicians has grown through the centuries from incidental wall decoration to an exhibition of national and international significance.

References

1. R. VAN MARLE, *Iconographie de l'art profane au Moyen-Age et à la Renaissance et la décoration des demeures*, I, La Haye 1931, pp. 13–17; H. KELLER, 'Die Entstehung des Bildnisses am Ende des Hochmittelalters', *Römisches Jahrbuch für Kunstgeschichte* III, 1939, pp. 227–356, especially p. 250.
2. KELLER, *op.cit.*, p. 251.
3. R. L. POOLE, *Catalogue of Portraits in the possession of the University, Colleges, City, and County of Oxford*, II, Oxford 1925, p. 9; E. CROFT-MURRAY, *Decorative Painting in England 1537–1837*, I, London 1962, p. 15.
4. O. MILLAR, *The Tudor, Stuart and Early Georgian Pictures in the Collection of Her Majesty the Queen*, London 1963, pp. 9–10, 50–51.
5. CROFT-MURRAY, *op.cit.*, pp. 15, 176.
6. R. VAN LUTTERVELT, 'Bijdrage tot de Iconographie van de Graven van Holland, naar aanleiding van de beelden uit de Amsterdamse Vierschaar', *Oud-Holland* LXXII, 1957, pp. 73–91, 139–159, 218–234.
7. MILLAR, *op. cit.*, pp. 9–10, 49–53.
8. KELLER, *op.cit.*, p. 251.
9. H. SCHROEDER, *Der Topos der Nine Worthies in Literatur und bildender Kunst*, Göttingen 1971.
10. TH. E. MOMMSEN, 'Petrarch and the decoration of the Sala virorum illustrium in Padua', *The Art Bulletin* XXXIV, 1953, pp. 95–116.
11. E. MICHEL, *Catalogue raisonné des peintures du moyen-âge, de la renaissance et des temps modernes, Peintures flamandes du XVe et du XVIe siècle, Musée National du Louvre*, Paris 1953, pp. 146–151.
12. R. L. MODE, 'Masolino, Uccello and the Orsini "Uomini Famosi"', *The Burlington Magazine* CXIV, 1972, pp. 369–378.
13. E. MÜNTZ, 'Le Musée de portraits de Paul Jove. Contributions pour servir à l'iconographie du Moyen Age et de la Renaissance', *Mémoires de l'Institut National de France, Académie des inscriptions et belles-lettres* XXXIII, 1901, pp. 249–343; J. ALAZARD, *Le portrait*

florentin de Botticelli à Bronzino, Paris 1938, pp. 221–224; P. O. RAVE, 'Paolo Giovio und die Bildnisviten-Bücher des Humanismus', *Jahrbuch der Berliner Museen* I, 1959, pp. 119–154.

14. MÜNTZ, *op.cit.*, pp. 264–270; ALAZARD, *op.cit.*, pp. 222–224; F. KENNER, 'Die Porträt-sammlung des Erzherzogs Ferdinand von Tirol', *Jahrbuch der Kunsthistorischen Sammlungen des Allerhöchsten Kaiserhauses* XIV, 1892, pp. 37–186; XV, 1893, pp. 147–259; XVII, 1896, pp. 101–274; XVIII, 1897, pp. 135–261; XIX, 1898, pp. 6–146; H. SCHWINDRAZHEIM, 'Eine Porträtsammlung Wilhelms IV, von Hessen und der "Güldene Saal" ', *Marburger buch für Kunstwissenschaft* X, 1937, 263–306.

15. RAVE, *op.cit.*, pp. 150–152.

16. RAVE, *op.cit.*, pp. 148–149.

17. KENNER, *op.cit.*; SCHWINDRAZHEIM, *op.cit.*

18. R. STRONG, *The English Icon; Elizabethan & Jacobean Portraiture*, London-New York 1969, pp. 45–46.

19. A. JANDA-BUX, 'Die Entstehung der Bildnissammlung an der Universität Leipzig und ihre Bedeutung für die Geschichte des Gelehrtenporträts', *Wissenschaftliche Zeitschrift der Karl-Marx-Universität. Wissenschaftliche Zeitschrift der Friedrich-Schiller-Universität. Gesellschafts- und Sprachwissenschaftliche Reihe* iv, 1954–1955, pp. 143–168; A. JANDA-BUX, 'Katalog des Kunstbesitzes der Universität Leipzig', *ibidem*, pp. 169–197; D. KUSCH, 'Die Rektoren- und Professorenbildnisse des 16. Jahrhunderts in der Friedrich-Schiller-Universität Jena. *Gesellschafts- und Sprachwissenschaftliche Reihe*, VII, 1957–1958, pp. 9–32; R. SCHOLL, *Die Bildnissammlung der Universität Tübingen 1477 bis 1927*, Stuttgart 1927.

20. E. HULSHOFF POL, 'The Library', *Leiden University in the seventeenth century. An Exchange of Learning*, Leiden 1975, pp. 416, 446; R. E. O. EKKART, 'Portraits in Leiden University Library', *Quaerendo* v, 1975, pp. 52–65, especially p. 58.

21. EKKART, *op.cit.*: *Icones Leidenses. De portretverzameling van de Rijksuniversiteit te Leiden*, Leiden 1973.

22. POOLE, *op.cit.*: J. W. GOODISON, *Catalogue of Cambridge Portraits, I, The University Collection*, Cambridge 1955; L. CUST, 'On portraits at the Universities', *Fasciculus Ioanni Willis Clark dicatus*, Cantabrigiae 1909, pp. 423–437.

23. POOLE, *op.cit.*, I, pp. x–xx, 1–130.

24. J. N. L. MYRES, 'The painted frieze in the picture gallery', *The Bodleian Library Record* III, 1950–1951, pp. 82–91; J. N. L. MYRES, 'Thomas James and the painted frieze', *ibidem* IV, 1952–1953, pp. 30–51; J. N. L. MYRES and E. C. ROUSE, 'Further notes on the painted frieze and other discoveries in the Upper Reading Room and the Tower Room', *ibidem* V, 1954–1956, pp. 290–308.

25. See Catalogue, I, 1964, p. 459.

26. Ditto, p. 463.

27. Ditto, p. 463; G. CLARK, *A History of the Royal College of Physicians of London*, Oxford I, 1964, p. 332 and pl. XIII.

28. See Catalogue, I, 1964, pp. 460–461.

29. POOLE, *op.cit.*, I, XI and Nos. 123, 126, 145, 149, 159, 166, 191; one painting has dis-appeared (p. 130).

30. POOLE, *op.cit.*, I, No. 252.

31. CLARK, *op.cit.*, II, 1964, pp. 534–535.

32. D. PIPER, *Catalogue of seventeenth-century Portraits in the National Portrait Gallery 1625–1714*,

Cambridge 1963, pp. 133–134.

33. W. R. LeFanu, *A Catalogue of the Portraits and other Paintings, Drawings and Sculpture in the Royal College of Surgeons of England*, Edinburgh-London 1960.

34. A so-called portrait of Thomas Linacre.

35. The only exception is Sir James Alderson (President 1867–1871).

36. 48 at the beginning of the century, 305 at the end.

37. A. M. Cooke, *A History of the Royal College of Physicians of London*, III, Oxford 1972, p. 1000.

38. T. R. Cullinan, 'The Statues of Harvey, Linacre and Sydenham', *Royal College of Physicians of London. College Commentary.* V, 1970–1971, pp. 17–19; Cooke, *op.cit.*, p. 843.

39. A. H. Driver, *Catalogue of Engraved Portraits in the Royal College of Physicians of London*, London 1952.

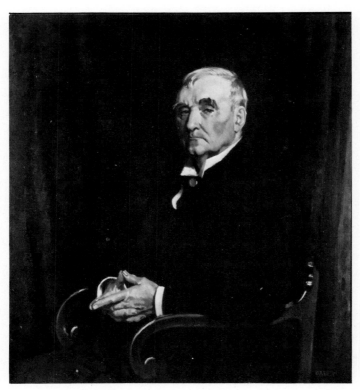

Fig. 1. David Lloyd-Roberts

*Take the face of a physician**

With special reference to the portraits in the College

David Piper

The face of the physician. This title, begotten by necessity on an unbegotten lecture, may mislead. It is not my aim to demonstrate that there are certain elements in the architecture of a physician's face that can be analysed and described in a codified form, from which any observer will be able to deduce, without prior knowledge, that a given face confronting him must be that of a physician. It sounds fairly absurd now even to suggest such an idea, but in fact the pursuit of it in the past, and the not-so-far-off past at that, has absorbed the energies of learned and ingenious men. In the early nineteenth century that eminent physiologist, Sir Charles Bell, believed that certain habits of facial expression, which could be formed, for example, from the specialised routines of a profession, could bring about structural changes in the facial tissues. Later Sir Francis Galton and then Karl Pearson had a go at this theme. Galton tried to precipitate the archetypal faces of various professions by superimposing a considerable number of photographs of faces of men in one profession one on top of the other; the final outline left on the paper should give the average face. The result alas proves generally to be a sort of bland anonymous map of no one in particular. The most recent general book on the Human Face, by John Liggett, in discussing this problem, reproduces a number of faces of men and invites his reader to deduce from them what their owner's professions are; apart from the faces I knew beforehand, I found I got most of them wrong. In passing though I might remark that Doctors are amongst the few who can, by their training, and habitually do, arrive at detailed specific and demonstrable conclusions from the study of individual human faces. Diagnosis, in fact – but the diagnosis is in terms of disease rather than that of the character of a human being.

It is not then the physician's face, in the literal and limited meaning of the word, that I wish to discuss, but more the whole face, the brave front of the whole physical persona, that the physician has presented to a sceptical public through the centuries

* Delivered at the Royal College of Physicians on 4 December 1974.

covered by the portraits in the College's collection. To attempt to prove there is a physician's face is vain; if there were such a thing it would mean for example that if you had the wrong kind of face you couldn't become a physician. But I think it is clear that there is, in any period, a stereotype, or a number of stereotype images, that hover, if in an often fairly generalised way, in the consciousness of the general public; images that they feel the physician ought to match more or less. These stereotypes modulate as fashions change, but there are various qualities that remain fairly constant.

But let me come to specifics. To start with, it seems only proper, in gratitude and piety, to take the Founder of these lectures. David Lloyd-Roberts was born in 1855, son of a cotton spinner, and began work by serving in a chemist's shop. Then, via an apprenticeship to the Professor of Physiology at Owens College, he proceeded to qualify. He became a Fellow in 1878, but he was always primarily associated with Manchester and especially St Mary's Hospital for Women and Children. He was a gynaecologist, and a distinguished one. But he was a man of many parts. Besides works on his own branch of medicine, he wrote on Dante and edited Sir Thomas Browne's *Religio Medici*. He was a collector of beautiful things – engravings, water-colours, glass, porcelain and so on, and also a bibliophile who, when he died in 1920 at the age of 85, left his library to the College, and also endowed this annual lecture. Sir William Orpen's portrait of him (Fig. 1) was commissioned by the College three years after his death, in 1923, but it is a replica of one that Orpen painted in 1915 and which is now at Manchester. Orpen was one of the most successful portrait painters of his time, celebrated for the brilliance and briskness of his attack on his sitters, and for his production of them as if in almost theatrical limelight, so that they can seem almost to start out of the canvas: the more picturesque the appearance in life of his sitters, the better he succeeded, even if he left himself open in some works to criticisms of slickness and even vulgarity. But his image of Lloyd-Roberts is a good and characteristic example: within the decorum of a presentation portrait, formal, an entirely traditional composition, yet enlivened by the gesture of the hands, that convinces as characteristic of the sitter, and by the bold and forthright capturing of the expression of the face. The corners of the mouth may be down – fairly unusual in portraits – but any impression of severity or melancholy seems offset by the eyes, perhaps most by the eyebrows. A slightly hooded but keen and scanning steady gaze. The prognosis, one feels, may not necessarily be favourable, but it will at least encourage one to die with decorum, like a gentleman, knowing one is in good hands.

It is then a face that well becomes a physician. But I doubt if it's true that if you didn't already know its owner was a physician, you would guess him to be so. The face would equally become, say, a distinguished admiral in mufti – those splendid eyebrows, perhaps, hoary with a glint of salt. In fact they have a close family re-semblance to the eyebrows of one of the most famous admirals of the time, Jackie Fisher. Still, overall, the image fits. I would think a stereotype of what a prosperous physician of the age would do well to look like. His dress, for example. Recently I found Lord Clark, in his autobiography, describing someone, about this time, as being like 'a Harley Street gout specialist, with purple stock and a cameo tie pin'. Here, black tie or stock, but the image of the whole man, that Kenneth Clark's two details summon up, corresponds very well.

The general point that one can draw from this, and that applies fairly consistently throughout the College's collection of portraits, is that physicians, in their daily confrontation with life, are sartorial conformists, discreet and conservative, tending indeed to the oldfashioned in their dress. Because, of course, they have to be, for they have to personify comfort and confidence to worried people; if a Fellow of the College were to bound into his consulting room geared up like the lead singer in a pop group, the confidence of a very large proportion of his patients would be severely shaken. In the portraits in the College, the impression of grave respectability is strengthened by the function the portraits were designed to serve: a considerable proportion of them, like this one, have a double role – to celebrate in the image of the individual a benefaction whether of goods or of services rendered, and through the benefaction the enduring virtue of the institution. This portrait was commissioned, in gratitude, by the College: many others have been commissioned likewise, or given by admirers. In such portraits those who commission them, their sitters, and their artists all naturally and amiably agree on a solution aimed to present the sitter composed at his best for posterity. So that glimpses of the physician actually at work, or even slightly dishevelled by the harassment of the doctor's normal round, are rare.

Here is another stereotype, of Lloyd-Roberts's generation, if a decade or so earlier than Lord Clark's comment. This is about 1890:

'If a gentleman walks into my rooms smelling of chloroform, with a black mark of nitrate of silver upon his right forefinger, and a bulge in the side of his top hat to show where he has secreted his stethoscope, I must be dull indeed if I do not pronounce him to be an active member of the medical profession ...'

That is of course Conan Doyle – himself a qualified and practising physician – alias Sherlock Holmes, diagnosing the dazzled Dr Watson's vocation. But smells elude the portrait painter; black marks on finger are normally washed off before the sitter takes the studio chair; and Lloyd-Roberts's glossy top hat, far less one with a workaday bulge, was evidently not considered a necessary attribute.

Before I leave Lloyd-Roberts there are a couple more thoughts that his image provokes. One – the eyebrows again perhaps – that despite the physician's traditional external respectability, a degree of personal eccentricity is permissible. This can arise from sheer sticking to tradition. Lloyd-Roberts used to clip clop about the shining raining streets of Manchester in full fig of a grand brougham long after such vehicles had gone out of fashion. Then there's the glint of a slightly sardonic wit in that facade – after all, he was wont to say of his chosen vocation that gynaecology embraced anything 'either curable or lucrative'. Lucrative his career certainly was

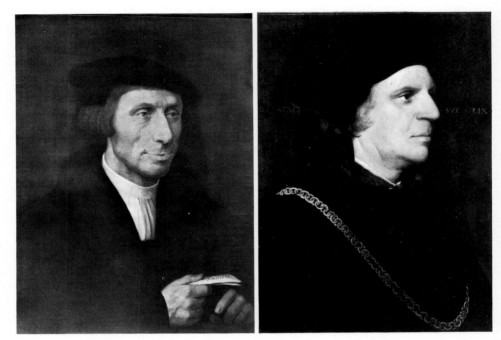

Fig. 2. Linacre   *Fig. 3.* Butts

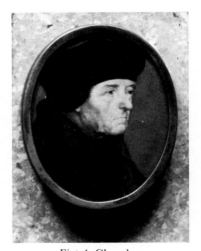

Fig. 4. Chambre

and that is not a-typical of many physicians though happily often allied with an endlessly open availability to poor as well as rich. It is though an important constituent in the nourishment of another quality that is surprisingly often found in successful physicians: an eager appetite for the arts, which itself has often in English society been considered as mildly if not wildly eccentric. Some of the most important collectors and patrons in English history are to be found in the physicians' ranks. Sir Hans Sloane, that well-known Chelsea practitioner, was virtually the founder of the British Museum itself; to the Hunter brothers, John and William, we owe two quite extraordinary collections, in the Royal College of Surgeons and in the Hunterian Museum at Glasgow – and there were many others, amongst them Lloyd-Roberts himself.

I must now though turn your attention to the collection as a whole, or rather to select a few but representative elements in it that illustrate the way in which physicians through the centuries have confronted English society. For the first century of the College's foundation, after 1518, there is almost nothing original: this is to be expected for it was only in the second half of the sixteenth century that the habit of portraiture became at all widespread in the professional classes, and only right at the end of the century that the institutional habit of commemorating founders or benefactors began to form. There are, though, three portraits I would like to mention – all copies, and relatively very late additions to the collection. First the Founder himself, a very desirable commodity in all piety: Thomas Linacre. This was painted by an obviously unusually talented College Beadle, Mr Miller, in 1810, and is copied from a painting in the Royal Collection. Like Lloyd-Roberts's, this is a face that certainly would do no discredit to the profession, though it is not in any way demonstrable as necessarily a physician's face. Still very vital and alert after four and a half centuries. But whether it really is Linacre one simply doesn't know: the attachment of Linacre's name to the original seems to have been made by about 1734, and why on earth christen it Linacre if there was no evidence for it? The doubt rests in the date inscribed on the paper in his hand. Mr Miller read it as 1521, and that, although the Netherlandish origin is certainly a bit awkward, would be quite compatible, as Linacre then was alive and well (he died in 1524); unfortunately recent cataloguers read the date on the original as 1527 or 1537 – if somewhat hesitant, they are united in *not* reading it as 1521.

But whether it is or it isn't, this can be accepted as giving a reasonable notion of what a physician might have looked like in the first half of the sixteenth century. Two others are a little bit later, early 1540s: Dr Butts and Dr Chambre. These are both copies after Holbein: Butts, by George Richmond some time before 1880, from the original in the Isabella Gardner Museum at Boston; Chambre a very beautiful copy in miniature by Peter Oliver, around 1620, from the original now in Vienna – very likely this is Oliver's miniature that is known to have belonged to Charles I. Both in the fairly sombre, if opulently sombre, garb associated with clerics, and it was of course via the church that most men of any kind of learning began their careers. Linacre was ordained; so was Chambre. Chambre was likewise a founding father of the College in 1518, while Butts became a Fellow in 1529. Neither of them appears to have played much part in the early history of the College, but both these portraits derive in fact from an institutional group-portrait, the earliest such in England, Holbein's painting of Henry VIII presenting their charter to the Barber-Surgeons. Here in the figure of Henry VIII, an oversize almost Byzantine idol, is feudal monarchy presiding over its servant profession of medicine. Whether the profession would perform such mass obeisance now may be doubted, but in Henry VIII's time it was only realistic. Chambre – here seen in his early 70s – reached an age, 88, remarkable in that time, and perhaps especially so in the case of men who were – as both Butts and Chambre were – very close to that very lethal monarch. Chambre you will note has probably lost most of his teeth, a hazard to which medical men are now less prone. But in the cases of Holbein's original versions of both portraits I think we have unusual evidence of the early interest of physicians in patronage: both, I think, were almost certainly repeats, ordered by the sitters for themselves, of their images as first shown in the group-portrait.

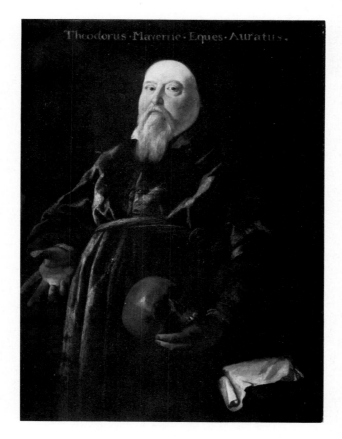

30

Fig. 5.
Sir Theodore de Mayerne

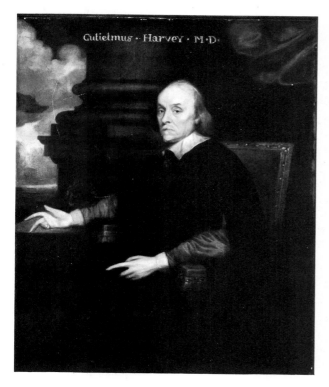

Fig. 6. William Harvey

Of the profession under Elizabeth the College has no originals, but it was towards the end of her reign, in 1596, that the College passed a strange Statute to which I don't know any exact parallel. It was then ordained that any Fellow (and indeed apparently any outsider) could hoist his own portrait or coat-of-arms on payment of £10. Presumably a fund-raising exercise though offering gravely unprofessional opportunities for self-advertisement: if anyone acted on it, it seems probable that the results were destroyed with so much else when the College building in Amen Corner burnt in the Great Fire of 1666. From that fire only two portraits were salvaged. There is however one rather splendid image of an earlier date that has survived because it came to the College only about 1688 after the Fire: Sir Theodore de Mayerne became the leading court physician under James I and Charles I – a Fellow in 1616. Sighted here in the College portrait (Fig. 5), by an unknown painter of considerable if fairly coarse Carravagesque power, perhaps in the 1630s and in agreeably informal wear, skull-cap and, almost, dressing-gown. I think though, that as he truly looks, he was an eccentric in the physicians' ranks, and as such, *qua* patient, I feel might have lacked confidence. Although a scientist of some original invention, he was also, although he must have known Harvey well, of the older times. Thus a balm for hypochondria, a Balsam of Bats for hypochondria: featuring as ingredients, adders, bats, sucking whelps, earth worms, hog's grease, the marrow of 31 a stag and the thigh bone of an ox ... But on second thoughts, for hypochondria, possibly indeed effective shock-treatment. In this portrait though he is demonstrated as a member of the profession by a rudimentary method that can be seen applied in many later medical portraits – by being given a medical attribute. Here a skull, and although this, in Elizabethan portraiture especially, appears often in lay portraits as a *memento mori*, it is here, it has been suggested, judging from the marks on the skull, introduced with specific reference to Mayerne's innovations in dissection of the skull. Perhaps not actual dissections – an ingredient in his gout powder was 'raspings of a human skull unburied'. De Mayerne again had a close connection with art and artists: he was interested in the chemistry of their pigments, and a large manuscript volume of his recordings of these survives in the British Museum. He sat to Rubens, probably twice, and it is only surprising that no evidence of a sitting to Van Dyck has yet emerged. He also collected cookery recipes; recommended a monthly excess of wine and food as a fine stimulant to the system – but died himself, alas, from drinking bad wine.

His almost exact contemporary, the great William Harvey, was of course a very different creature. Whether, from my point of view as potential patient, he would have inspired more confidence must be uncertain. 'Not tall' – this part of John Aubrey's account from long personal knowledge – 'Not tall, but of the lowest stature, round faced, olivester complexion: little eie, round, very black, full of spirit ... very cholerique and in his young days wore a dagger; but the Dr. would be too apt to draw out his dagger upon every slight occasion.' No man for a patient to argue with, and also full of disquieting if brilliant innovations – patients tend to be conservative in their ideas about treatment as doctors do in their dress. The chief portrait of Harvey in the College – and probably the most famous of all – is a sober celebration of a presiding genius, in what was already a traditional formula (Fig. 6). Three-quarter length, seated, in his black gown and holding his doctoral hat, his social status demonstrated as armigerous by his coat of arms on the base of the pillar. It was probably commissioned by the College, whom Harvey served so well, and it is one of those two portraits salvaged from the fire of 1666 – perhaps damaged then, and the sad work of a restorer in Harvey's right hand is only too visible. There is a hint of apotheosis in the pillar, the swirling drape, and the sky beyond, but these are conventional baroque props borrowed from Van Dyck; it is really a modest picture, though the outstretched hand may once, before it was damaged, have conveyed an immemorial gesture, implying almost: *Si monumentum requiris, circumspice*. For the extraordinary genius that inhabited the body, it is of course inadequate, but then how adequate was the body itself? It underlines the perpetual dilemma of the portrait painter, expressed in another way by Max Beerbohm when he complained that so few people look like themselves. In the case of truly seminal geniuses, succeeding generations have sometimes tended, when they find the contemporary portrait inadequate, to revise it more in accordance with their own idea of what it ought to look like, and I shall have a brief glance at the revisions of Harvey later.

32

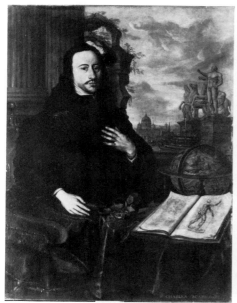

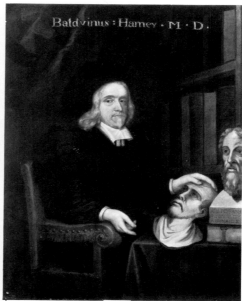

Fig. 7. Sir Charles Scarburgh

Fig. 8. Baldwin Hamey

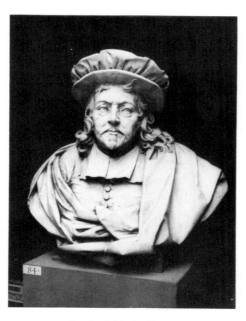

Fig. 9. Baldwin Hamey

33

In the new building designed by Robert Hooke for the College in Warwick Lane, after 1666, the portraits began to accumulate mainly by gift, and a number of portraits of this period have in fact been acquired relatively recently. Most of the as-it-were standard formal head-and-shoulders portraits of the period are not of great artistic quality, nor very revealing about their subjects. But they do incidentally preserve beside the wraiths of their subjects, examples of the work of several minor but very rare artists, and they include some very fascinating documents.

Sir Charles Scarburgh, for example, first physician to Charles the II: a very strange, allusive and romantic portrait, perhaps by a very little known Dutch painter called Jean Demetrius, in the 1650s. His major interest, as physician, is signalled clear enough by the volume of Vesalius open at Book 2, plate 2. The gold watch, the zodiacal globe, the prisms, hint at the virtuoso, the elegant man of curious learning, and specifically at his interest in mathematics. But why it is sited in Rome, with that view past the sculptured horsemen on the Quirinal to St Peter's, remains an enigma and as such perhaps adds to the potency of this mysterious image – this very erect, rather brooding figure all in black with the ruined arch and the cloud-charged sky behind, even though the artist's command of perspective was, to put it mildly, a bit rum. Further compounding the enigma is the relationship, also mysterious but certainly there, between the portrait and one by Van Bemmell now in the Hunterian at Glasgow, of Harvey himself likewise with a long view over Rome. What shared classical nostalgia the two men, who were close and long friends, had, we do not know.

Scarburgh appears again in a small 19th century water-colour copy of a painting by Richard Greenbury that still belongs to the Barber Surgeons, painted perhaps in the 1640s. Very rare in English painting – the portrayal of an anatomy demonstration, and I suspect *not* a very literal representation: even then Scarburgh and his colleague, Dr. Aris, would hardly have performed in such full fig, doctorally hatted and voluminously gowned. It is a strange but quaint document, all the quainter in contrast with the most famous exercise on this theme, painted by Rembrandt in Holland about the same time, of Dr Tulp demonstrating. Another document, almost as naive, though rather later, records one of the College's greatest benefactors, Baldwin Hamey the Younger, painted in 1674 by the very, and understandably, obscure painter, Snelling: but in its way it's rather charming. Again in black gown and puffed doctoral hat, seated in his study, with his loyalties personified in the shape of two busts, one (that almost slipping off the table) of Hippocrates, the other inscribed in Greek with the unexpected and unexplained name of Aristophanes. That was a later gift to the College, which had already served its benefactor much better by commissioning from the sculptor Edward Pierce what proved to be one of the finest English portrait busts of the seventeenth century – at once monumental and quick with the conviction of an individual likeness.

The fashion in England for portrait busts – other than in funeral monument sitings in churches – started generally much later than this, but the College seems to have had a precocious appreciation of sculpture. A life-size statue of Harvey was there

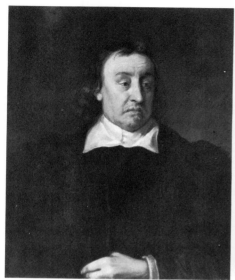

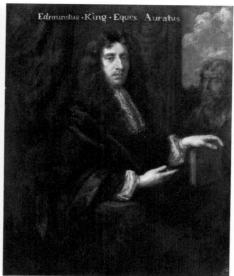

Fig. 10. Sir Francis Prujean

Fig. 11. Sir Edmund King

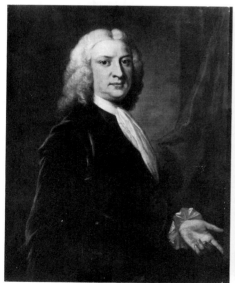

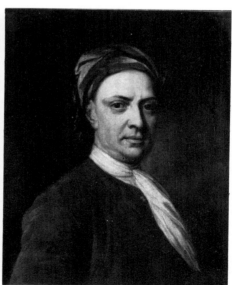

Fig. 12. Peter Shaw

Fig. 13. Peter Shaw

35

before the fire and perished in it: two more statues, of Charles II and Sir John Cutler, were ordered for the new building and survive in the Guildhall Museum. The splendid bust of Hamey though now constitutes a challenge to some pious benefactor – it needs cleaning and also needs proper mounting. We have the sculptor's first thoughts as to how he meant it to look, in a drawing in the Ashmolean Museum: the conception altered as the bust progressed, but with that drawing as guide one should be able to produce a more worthy setting than it has at the moment.

In painting this – late seventeenth and early eighteenth century – was a conformist age. There are some exceptions – Dr Prujean is one, by a painter called Robert Streater in 1662. He's known almost solely as a large scale mural decorator, but on the evidence of this brilliantly idiosyncratic characterisation one wishes Streater had done more. There is nothing though either in the face or elsewhere here that refers to the sitter's profession, unless that vivid expression of fastidious melancholy be considered an occupational trait. Prujean again was a man much interested in the arts, a collector of pictures and a virtuoso on rare musical instruments. Much more characteristic of the time are portraits like that of Sir Edmund King, who attended Charles II in his terminal illness: very grand, very good as a late work of the leading court painter, Sir Peter Lely, about 1680. Yet even though identified as of the profession – the bust of Hippocrates again presiding – the characterisation is that of an elegant gentleman, and the baroque style, with its love of movement, of broad sweeps of draping and colour, somewhat extinguishes the individuality of the sitter. So too does the wig, here first seen in full splendour: the wig, stylistically, accords with the baroque need for voluminous movement, but it far outlasted the baroque period, continuing in various forms from around 1660 to nearly 1800. For almost a century and a half, almost all men of sense – and this period embraced the age of reason – cut off their hair in order to wear someone else's. In one portrait in the College Dr Peter Shaw does it in a form popular some sixty years later, about 1740, but a second portrait of him shows him in informal leisure wear: he has taken off his wig, but in order to protect his naked, perhaps shaven, head from notorious English draughts he has to put on instead a kind of turban night-cap. And though the wig in the first portrait is much less concealing than in the portrait of King, one can see here how much more strongly the features of the face tell in the wig-less portrait. Both are primarily the portrait of a gentleman of social standing: neither refers to Dr Shaw's medical calling. In another portrait of a medical gentleman (Fig. 14), the sitter is displayed as such – again a fascinating exercise by a very rare painter, the most baroque of English-born painters, one Edmund Lilley, about 1695. A specimen of the wig floribundissimus: the doctor's hat sitting on it rather uncertainly, the robes and hood of presumably a Cambridge M.D. taken full advantage of: the specific allusion of the pen and the document, if there was one, is lost. The sitter, Edward Tyson, was in fact one of the most brilliant of early comparative anatomists.

36   The case of Dr Richard Mead offers an unusual opportunity of surveying the

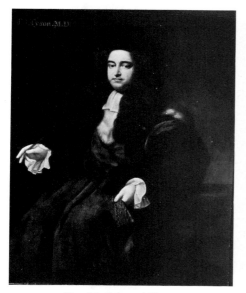

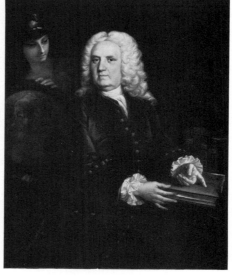

Fig. 14. Edward Tyson   *Fig. 15.* Richard Mead

variety of solutions the portrait artist might achieve in the mid-eighteenth century. Professionally, he was a fabulous success: George II's physician, with an income equivalent to at least sixty or seventy thousand pounds today. A voracious collector of books and works of art: an active patron. He is celebrated in the history of art not only as perhaps the greatest English collector of works of art in his time (Sir Hans Sloane's interests were more in the field of science), but as the physician to whom Watteau turned in a last vain search for cure from tuberculosis, and Mead had two paintings by Watteau. He is celebrated in many places by his memorial portrait, not only in the Royal College, but in the National Portrait Gallery, the Bodleian, the Foundling Hospital and the Royal Society. The formal memorial portrait that the College owns seems about 1740, but it could be a posthumous painting; Mead died in 1754. It places him very firmly in his professional context: the full wig, the brown velvet coat; on the table volumes of Galen, Hippocrates and Celsus, with a paper inscribed with his name, *Dr Mead*; on the left, held by a figure of Minerva presiding like a muse, homage to his more recent spiritual ancestry – a shield or plaque bearing a profile of William Harvey. Two of the other portraits of Mead in the College are in startling contrast – variations on a theme, by one Arthur Pond. The existence of two versions is strange, for this portrait design seems certainly not to have been approved by its subject. Pond in fact issued an etching of it in 1739, inscribed probably sardonically *Non sibi sed toti* (not for himself but for all); a mezzotint was also published. But a contemporary observer recorded some fuss – 'a profil, drawn and etched by Mr Pond in the manner of Rinebrandt very like the Doctor but when done, being in short ruff-hair – no wig etc. The Doctor particularly desired

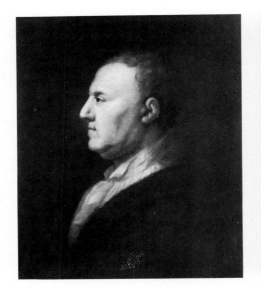

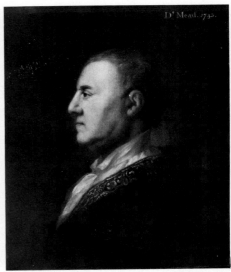

Fig. 16. Richard Mead   *Fig. 17.* Richard Mead

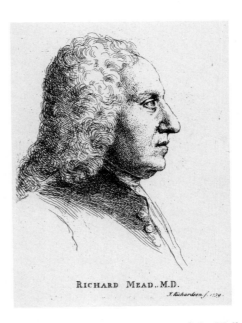

         Fig. 18. Richard Mead (Reproduced by courtesy of the Wellcome Trustees)

Mr Pond to suppress it, / from whence this proceeded the Doctor would not give any answer nor reason / one may easily guess, that it appears like an old mumper, as Rhinebrandt's heads usually do. / Such works give pleasure to virtuosi; but not to the Publick Eye of the nice part of human nature (and modish people) and it is not the true characteristic of a fine gentleman as Dr Mead always appears / therefore in pictures it is a false character – and debases the idea of a polite person –' But Pond, who was certainly a bit of a joker, did publish and one measure of the strength of the Doctor's feelings is probably an etching of himself by another artist, Richardson, published the same year, in 1739, and very likely as a counterblast (Fig. 18). The doctor is shown decently wigged. I suspect indeed the wig was particularly associated with the stereotype of the proper decorum to be observed by physicians – indeed, later, in 1778, you will find Boswell lamenting, diagnosing a 'General levity in the age', finding physicians in bag-wigs, a rather foppish frivolous variant not to be compared in dignity with the full bottom.

However, the comment of about 1740 that I have just quoted is a just analysis of the virtues of portraits as of their limitations, and it applies fairly consistently through-out the College's collections up to now. Most of us really would rather see the great men of the past informally, even if like an 'old mumper', but neither the sitters nor the institutions they represent tend to allow this. 'The idea' is 'of a polite person': Rembrandt is all right for art but not in polite society: the master of manners of the age, Lord Chesterfield, confirmed this: 'I love la belle Nature: Rembrandt paints caricatures'. It is easy enough to mock this now, but if you transform it into con-temporary terms you may get a shock: Francis Bacon has yet to paint a President of this Royal College.

I – and the artists – have still not quite done with Richard Mead. After his death, Askew commissioned a posthumous bust from the brilliant French sculptor Roubiliac (Fig. 19). It is in this form that the mid-eighteenth century really stated Mead's claim amongst the immortals, for by then the classicizing bust had become the accepted medium to celebrate heroes. The fashion answered the classicizing taste in architecture, marble busts in marble halls, and equated consciously the British heroes of today and yesterday with those of Greece and Rome. It was applied retrospectively: for Harvey by Scheemakers, actually presented by Mead himself to the College in 1739 and probably commissioned shortly before that (Fig. 20). Harvey happily in his British doublet, but Mead, as befits the formidable Roman head that would so well become some dignitary of the Roman republic, has the formal drapery that suggests a toga, and here the lack of wig is very far from suggesting an 'old mumper'. A few years later, perhaps to complete a quartet to preside over the Censors' Room, the College commissioned, in 1758, a retrospective bust from Joseph Wilton of Sydenham (Fig. 21). This is not so happy: a fine head if much idealised from the modest original painting, but the costume of 1660 misunderstood by the sculptor of a century later, and it – and the wig – rather awkwardly consorting with the hint of toga.

39

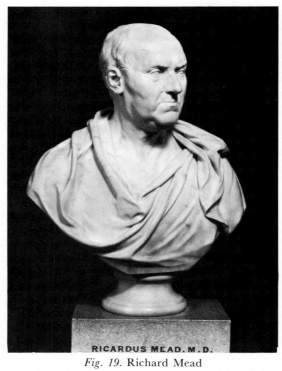

RICARDUS MEAD. M.D.

Fig. 19. Richard Mead

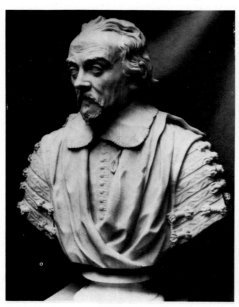

Fig. 20. William Harvey

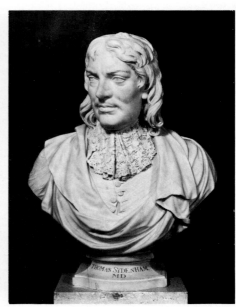

Fig. 21. Thomas Sydenham

40

In painting, the eighteenth century saw the consolidation of the tradition of recording the continuity of the College in the form of a sequence of portraits of succeeding Presidents, painted as Presidents. There is of course no Presidential face any more than there is a medical face, but there is perhaps a Presidential expression, of *gravitas*, a dignity and decorum becoming the presider, its specific relevance usually indicated by the President's robe. These portraits are inevitably formal, for they have to try to encapsulate the dignity and tradition of the institution within the image of the individual. The danger of course is of falling into a formula that suggests a fairly void and dead pomposity. Sir William Browne, President in 1765, in his portrait by Thomas Hudson is so pompous as to be both almost incredible and rather cherishable – but then Browne was in real life a masterpiece of absurdly ineffectual pomposity. He is certainly insisting here on status: in the President's gown, holding the Caduceus in one hand, the College Statutes in the other. You will note it is a wholelength – a rarity as such in the collection – but that the life-scale whole length need not be either pretentious or pompous is happily demonstrated by R.E. Pine's portrait of Dr Archer in 1782. This was painted not for the College but for the Inoculation Hospital, which is seen through the archway: it is a benign, most courteous image, retaining an engaging modesty and informality in spite of the quite elaborate contrivance of the composition with the colossal bust of Aesculapius with the traditional serpent twisted round its plinth. It seems entirely in character with

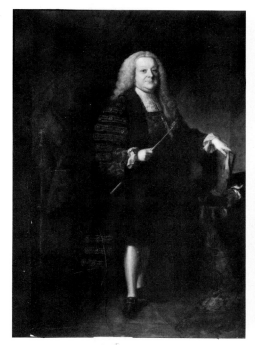
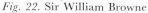

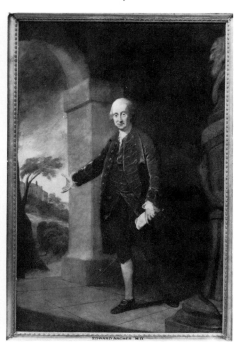

Fig. 22. Sir William Browne   *Fig. 23.* Edward Archer   41

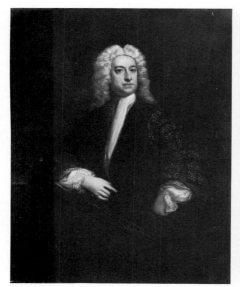 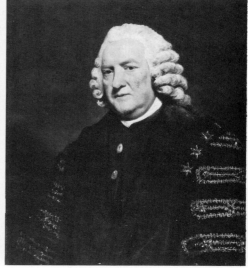

Fig. 24. Henry Plumptre   *Fig. 25.* William Pitcairn

the gentleman shown that when he died he made good by bequest to each of the Hospital Governors – who had paid for the portrait – each one's contribution of cash.

The comparison is a bit unfair as in the two decades between Hudson's painting of Browne and Pine's of Archer, a revolution in English portrait painting had consolidated itself, due largely to the genius of Sir Joshua Reynolds. The Presidential portrait of Henry Plumptre, President from 1740–45, is a decorous effigy in the style of Hudson. It was presented by the sitter. Whereas in Reynolds's painting of William Pitcairn, President from 1775 to 1785, you can see the admirable Reynolds's characteristic command of the atmospherics of individual life, a sense of the sitter being, not posed frozen for posterity, but still two hundred years later looking out on us as if poised between one movement and the next, one moment and the next. Pitcairn is no less a president than Plumptre, but it is to Pitcairn rather than Plumptre that I would go, in serene confidence, to unveil any of my more distressing and intimate ailments.

The College is fortunate in possessing a range of admirable informally formal portraits by artists of Reynolds's following, like Hoppner. But I'd rather for the moment inspect a couple of rare eccentricities. The first is still in Reynolds's orbit, the masterpiece of 1764 of a woman painter, Mary Black, though she may have had collaboration with her father Thomas, who seems to have worked in Reynolds's studio. The sitter wrote to Mary – 'Sure I was bedevilled to let you make your first attempt upon my gracefull person ... drawn like a Hog in armour, or a poor melancholy poet in a Garrett ... as good luck would have it your father has taken it

42

away to mend it or burn it'. He was Dr Messenger Monsey.

Monsey was an obscure if always fairly dotty country practitioner, until he got an emergency call to attend a rich London aristocrat. Evidently a successful attendance, for his patient translated him to London and prosperity, where he became a friend of people like Lord Chesterfield and David Garrick, and celebrated or notorious in London as one of the city's most picturesque eccentrics. In the College context, for which of course it was not commissioned, this portrait has an almost startlingly relaxed and domestic air. Even his spectacles are shown – the earliest in the College collection by some eighty years; in fact I think there's only one portrait until recently that shows a Fellow actually wearing his spectacles (Clendinning). Something of the same comfortableness is seen though in another great rarity, the only certain surviving work of a Chinese modeller called Chitqua, who was active in London for two or three years around 1770. It is of Anthony Askew (Fig. 27). He is formally robed in scarlet doctor's gown, and holding the College's famous gold-headed cane, but he sits his improbable chinoiserie rock seat with a nice blend of dignity, amiability and inscrutable if benevolent oriental expression lent him surely by the artist.

Both Askew and Monsey are still formally wigged; on the other hand their dress light tan colour in the one case, oyster-grey satin in the other – is far from sombre. Reverting to the more formal mode of portraiture, and looking on some fifty years, we find an entirely transformed presentation of the physician's person to the public. Sir Henry Halford, President between 1820 and 1844, was painted by the President of the Royal Academy, Sir Thomas Lawrence, in the 1820s (Fig. 28). His dress

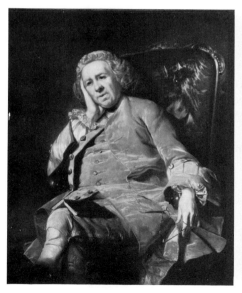

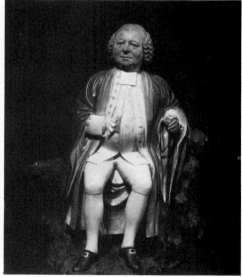

Fig. 26. Messenger Monsey   *Fig. 27.* Anthony Askew   43

reflects the revolution in male costume wrought in the Regency by Beau Brummell, which was essentially a withdrawal from what Brummell considered the garish motley of eighteenth-century polychrome finery into discreet, almost invisible but beautifully tailored black. 'A certain exquisite propriety' was how Byron defined the secret of Brummell's appearance, and from now on the physician will conform to such a sombre and *subfusc* propriety. Though the wig has gone, in fact Sir Henry is here a bit old-fashioned – subscribing still (perhaps as Court Physician) to knee-breeches, but Lawrence, the supreme visual interpreter of Regency elegance, has shown him far from sombre in his darks. Lawrence could highlight the radiance of keen intelligence in a handsome face as could no other, and this is the physician in his role of courtier, of aristocrat of intellect and achievement in his profession: the robe of the President of the College is draped not on his person but casually over the back of the chair, and the Star of Knight Commander of the Hanoverian Order on his breast shines all the more brightly. The theme is repeated, slightly more relaxed and in slightly less theatrical architectural setting, for Queen Adelaide's physician, Sir Charles Mansfield Clarke, by a close follower of Lawrence's, Samuel Lane, in 1832 (Fig. 29). Still knee-breeches, but the noble dome of the bald head making no concession to a toupé far less a wig. And then, twenty years on, in 1853, at last the stereotype of the successful Victorian metropolitan physician that was to endure with only small modifications till 1914, and perhaps even later. Another Clark, Sir James Clark: bald on top again, but compensating by cultivation of undergrowth lower down. Silk-faced frock-coat, trousers, gloves, and immaculate top hat, though with no trace of a stethoscope bulge (Fig. 30).

This image may reflect an early influence of photography, though it is indeed very early to do so, but the pose, perhaps the top hat too, do remind one very forcibly of the conventional studio photograph, and by 1850 the camera was just becoming sophisticated enough to record this sort of effect. I cannot here go into the complex history of give-and-take between photographer and artist in the nineteenth century, but one thing the camera did do was to give the public – and the artist – a yard-stick for the assessment of accurate rendering of detail. This applied sometimes even to the sculptors. The College owns a number of nineteenth century busts: many of them – it was an eclectic age – continue in the classical tradition of toga'ed marble, but sometimes the sculptor too felt impelled to aim at something like the detail of a 3-D photograph. That it is always successful, is doubtful. Through its classical associations, through its very medium, the portrait bust at its best seems as it were to distance its subject. Though it is, as in Roubiliac's Mead, capable of expressing considerable detail in a very lively fashion, it is also in a sense generalised and set apart, monochrome, and as it were a distillation of the sitter's essence from everyday ephemeral trivia, and demanding a niche or pedestal. Many Victorian exponents of the art tended to fall between two stools. George Simonds, for example, who conjured Arthur Leared out of marble in 1881 (Fig. 31). As I am sure Leared was, only in marble, and the idiom a bit odd – his frock coat and his gown faithfully

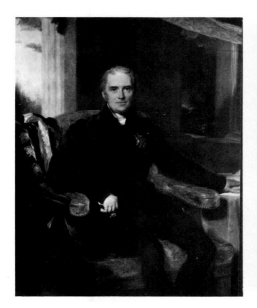

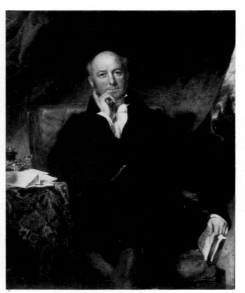

Fig. 28. Sir Henry Halford   *Fig. 29.* Sir Charles Mansfield Clarke

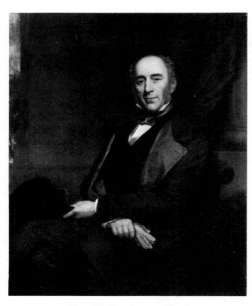

Fig. 30. Sir James Clark   45

rendered but cut off at the base rather unhappily, giving the impression that his hands are thrust into his invisible (marble) trousers. And really spectacular side-whiskers seem somehow difficult to marry into this artistic convention.

The retrospective celebration of past geniuses, by use of a classicizing bust, rather faded in the nineteenth century. The heroic attitude of the eighteenth century gave way, in the wake of the Romantic movement, to an interest in the authentic original, which also has something of the aura of a relic. But where the originals were scarce, the demand leads to supply – by fakes. The early nineteenth century is the boom period for forgery of Shakespeare portraits, and the College itself has one nineteenth century fake of Harvey. The Victorians though also went in a great deal for, not heroic so much as sentimental and anecdotal reconstruction of the heroes of the past, and the College has two Victorian images of Harvey, pleasant if perhaps uncharacteristically sweet for the subject. One is a painting by R. Hannah, 1848, of Harvey demonstrating perhaps the valves of a heart (not very clearly defined, but in an admirably clean handkerchief), to no less than Charles I himself, with plenty of picturesque detail around (Fig. 32). The other, a little terracotta statuette by C. B. Birch, of 1886, shows a highly idealised, almost saintly figure in meditation, again over a heart in his left hand. With the fawn recumbent between his legs, he might be a modern St Francis, unless of course it is from the fawn that he has plucked the heart (Fig. 33).

To revert to the main-stream: the output of professional portraits of medical men in Victorian times was considerable, and the blacks and greys of the professional uniform were often relieved by the rich colour of doctoral gowns. The most impressive portraits though are perhaps fairly sombre; for the portrait painters the example of Reynolds, of Titian and Van Dyck, tended to yield to enthusiasm for Velasquez, and this agreed fairly happily with the trend of Victorian elder statesmen – in all walks of life, not only politics – towards the ideal presentation of the self as a Grand Old Man. Two admirably forceful images of the kind: Sir Andrew Clark, President from 1888–1893, by Frank Holl in 1888, and Sir Richard Quain, Millais's last portrait, of 1896. Quain was incidentally, the personal physician of the Grand Old Man himself, Gladstone, and the aura of confident moral uprightness is very comparable.

That brings me in time almost to my starting point with David Lloyd-Roberts. Since then the College tradition of portraiture has continued, especially for Presidents, and has produced some admirable images. To choose from many, two fairly recent ones are the Epstein of Lord Brain and the Annigoni of Lord Moran. Epstein was a fairly revolutionary artist, Annigoni is firmly rooted in the traditions and techniques of the past. Both give a vivid equivalent of their sitters, though the Epstein may raise a few doubts. This century has seen an almost overwhelming interest in the purely formal rather than the representational values of art, an interest of course inimical to portraiture. Winston Churchill once maintained that any portrait should be at least 75% sitter, and not more than 25% artist: the artist now tends to claim much

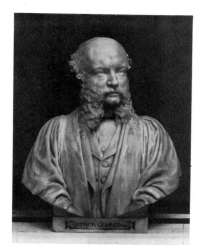

Fig. 31. Arthur Leared

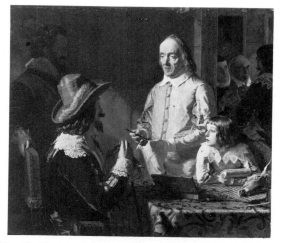

Fig. 32. Harvey demonstrating circulation to Charles I

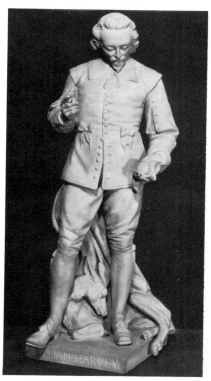

Fig. 33. William Harvey

47

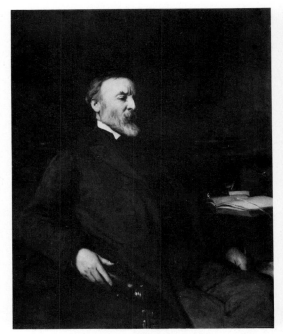

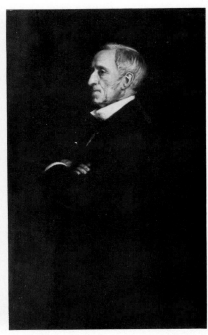

Fig. 34. Sir Andrew Clark　　　　　　　*Fig. 35.* Sir Richard Quain

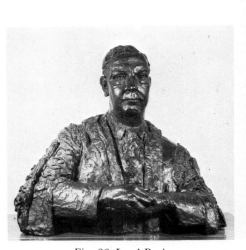

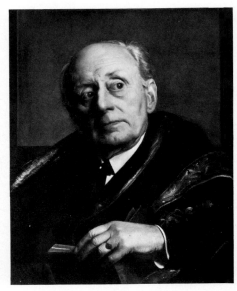

48　　　　　　*Fig. 36.* Lord Brain　　　　　　*Fig. 37.* Lord Moran of Manton

more, even – as in Picasso's most severe and pure cubist portraits – to the extent of obliterating the sitter entirely.

These remarks have been highly selective according to the space available; if they persuade one or two to look a bit closer at the College's portraits they will have served their purpose. I hope they have not seemed too peripheral, departing at tangents from their stated concern, the face, to matters like clothes, fashion, art. This is inevitable: the essence of each unique human face is precisely that it is unique, so that generalisations about it are by definition difficult to justify. But I would end by referring you to physicians' faces. Happily they are still worn by all physicians, and of course not stilled, as in portraits, but in action – the ever-changing register of the personality. As such, crucial in the dialogue between physician and patient. In 1656, the diarist John Evelyn was writing to his wife – 'Be careful of your face, my dear.' The same message applies still, perhaps even more to physicians than members of other professions.

The Portraits

with biographical notes by Gordon Wolstenholme and
descriptions by John F. Kerslake

Bertram Louis Abrahams 1870–1908 F. 1904

Only son of the headmaster of the Jews' Free School in Spitalfields, London. He had a brilliant career at University College and later was appointed to the Westminster Hospital.

Abrahams took a keen interest in the social welfare of his community and was a founder of the Jewish Lads' Brigade; he loved cricket, and enjoyed teaching – at which he excelled.

For years he was dogged by 'kidney trouble' and this persuaded him to find a warmer climate in Egypt. However, the disease resulted in his death at the early age of 38.

The Bertram Louis Abrahams Lectureship in Physiology was established in his memory at the Royal College of Physicians in 1941.

Oils on canvas, 30 by 24⅞ inches, by Solomon J. Solomon, 1908

Short half length, head slightly to right, hands not seen; smooth black hair, dark brown eyes, pince-nez, thick brown moustache on upper lip, cleft chin, sallow complexion; white wing collar, black tie and suit; dark green background, lit from the left. Inscribed on the stretcher: *B L ABRAHAMS / SOLOMON*

Presented by his daughter Miss Margery Abrahams, November 1970.

Not signed or dated, the date presumably being supplied by the donor. It appears to be the only recorded portrait and should not be confused with Solomon's three-quarter length of the sitter's father, L. B. Abrahams, headmaster of the Jews' Free School, Spitalfields, exhibited at the Royal Academy 1908.

Ref: R.A. catalogue 1908 (481); *Royal Academy Pictures*, 1908, p. 103, rep.; al. from Miss Abrahams, 7 June 1960; *Annals*, 28 January 1971, p. 12b.

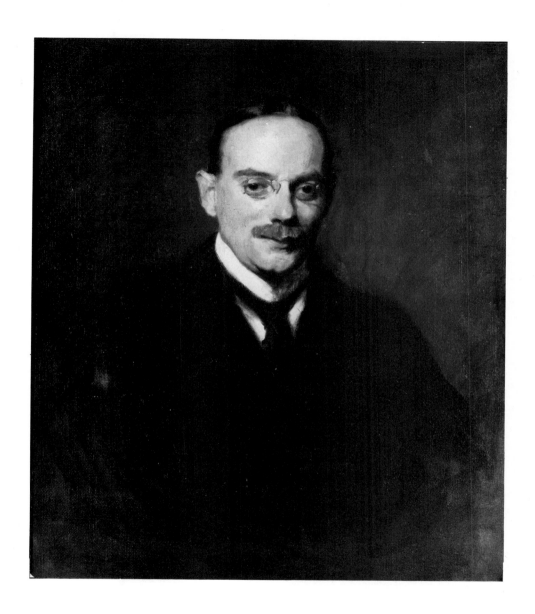

Anthony Addington 1713–1790 F. 1756

Physician and confidant to Lord Chatham, and in 1788 called in by the Prince of Wales to advise on the mental condition of George III.

(Catalogue I pp. 18–19)

2. Painting, oils on glass, 16¾ by 12⅜ inches, arched top, by John Rowell of Reading, c. 1750

Short half length, head to left, shoulders fronting spectator; brown eyes, plump face, slightly upturned nose, full bottom lip, double chin with slight cleft, short neck, youthful appearance; long brown wig, scarlet gown over coat and waistcoat, white lace cravat; light background, yellow spandrels.

Presented to the College by Dr. E. H. P. Cave (through Dr. K. Bryn Thomas) *c.* 1959. Removed from the stair-head of 73 London Street, Reading, which Addington built for himself *c.* 1748, opposite John Rowell's house.

Except for the coat and waistcoat which could be mid-eighteenth century, the costume would have been in fashion in the last decade of the seventeenth century. The scarlet gown, perhaps suggesting medicine, and the provenance of the piece are however in favour of the identification. The source of the portrait has not been identified. The only certain likeness is Banks' admirable bust of the sitter in old age, 1790/91. The attribution is given by Dr. Thomas of Reading, who notes similar work in the nearby churches of Harpsden and Arborfield.

Ref: Annals, 30 April 1959, p. 44s; *Catalogue*, I, 1964, pp. 18–19; Notes and news cutting in the R.C.P. Library; S. M. Gold, *John Rowell*, 1965, pp. 51–52; Information M. Archer, Esq., V. & A. Museum, 1975.

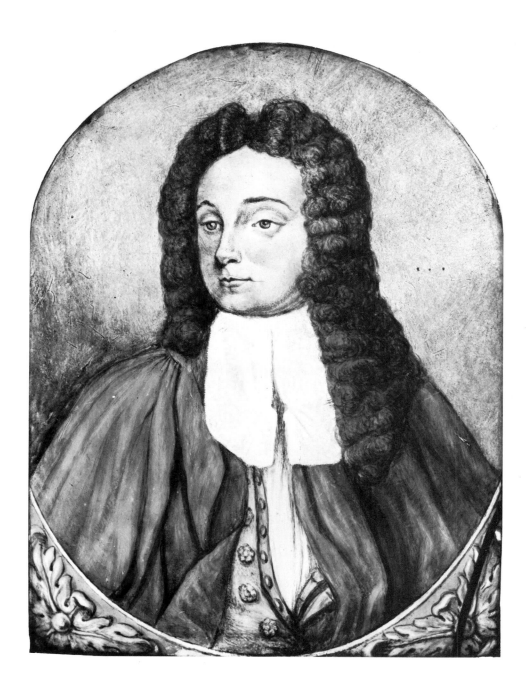

Prince Albert 1819–61

The child of a broken marriage, Prince Albert's upbringing was largely supervised by his two grandmothers. He did not care for women much and as a child resented their authority. Later, he was to find it difficult to adjust to the peculiar limbo of his position as Victoria's prince consort, and the British people certainly did not make things easy for him.

Albert applied himself with Germanic thoroughness to whatever he undertook and made a conscientious student. His passion in life was music, but he showed an interest in science as well as in the arts, and the International Exhibition of 1851 was his own idea. He was concerned that the character of the Queen's court should be above reproach – so much so that he himself never went anywhere without an equerry as chaperon. Victoria came to lean more and more heavily on him for his advice and moral strength. As father to the heir to the throne Albert emerges in an unsympathetic light – he expected so much of himself that he clearly expected too much of Edward – but as a husband he was worshipped, and even politicians who were at first suspicious of the role he played came to respect if not to like him.

Had he lived longer, a collision between Parliament and the monarchy would, it seems, have been inevitable, the prince being bent on more power for the throne, and his early death may even have averted revolution in this country. But, never physically tough, the standards the prince forced on himself soon wore him out and typhoid fever dealt the final death-blow when he was only 42.

Medallion by Timothy Butler, plaster, 35 ½ inches diameter, 1869

Head, profile to left; receding hair, moustache, side-whiskers; painted grey, within a gold rim; lettered above the head *ALBERT PRINCE CONSORT* and, below *BORN 1819 DIED 1861.*

Commissioned by the College, 1869.

The source of this image is not recorded but may well have been a bust like that by W. Theed 1862 in the Royal Society of Arts, or a photograph such as the widely circulated profile by J. E. Mayall of Regent Street, 1861. On the portraits of Albert see Ormond.

Ref: al. to the sculptor, settling his account for £8.18.6d., 20 November 1869; R. Ormond, *National Portrait Gallery Early Victorian Portraits*, I, 1973, pp. 13–15, II, pl. XIX.

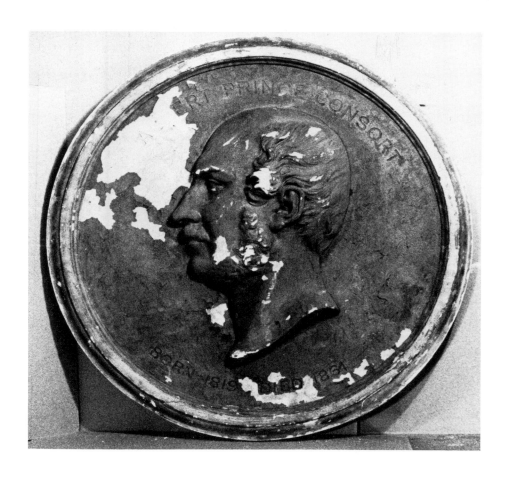

Basil William Sholto Mackenzie,
2nd Baron Amulree 1900– F. 1946

Only son of the 1st Baron Amulree whom he succeeded in 1942. Educated at Lancing College, and Gonville and Caius College, Cambridge, subsequently studying in Paris and at University College Hospital, London. He spent much of his early career as a medical officer in the Ministry of Health and was then appointed Physician to University College Hospital where he established a national reputation for his emphasis on the special care required by the elderly. The portrait was presented as a tribute to him by members of the British Geriatric Society, of which he was President. An elegant bachelor, Amulree is a familiar figure in the House of Lords where he has devoted much thought to problems of health care and the quality of medical education and practice, and where he has overcome a natural hesitancy in speech to play a leading role in debates on such subjects.

Oils on canvas, 36 by 28 inches, by Raymond Piper, 1966

Half length seated, slightly to right, hands clasped to table; white hair, deep blue eyes, fresh complexion; grey pin-stripe coat, white collar, white striped shirt, grey tie, gold monocle suspended on black cord; a lamp above his right shoulder, and on the wall behind a large earthenware plate, and the bottom of a framed picture. Signed and dated bottom left: *Raymond Piper '66.*

On indefinite loan from the sitter, to whom it was presented by the British Geriatric Society.

Painted in Lord Amulree's room; the chair in which he sits, the antique vase and the Picasso plate were among his favourite pieces. The sitter was photographed for the National Photographic Record in 1949, and 1963.

58   *Ref:* al. R. Piper, 12 March 1976 al. T. H. Howell, 20 Sept. 1975.

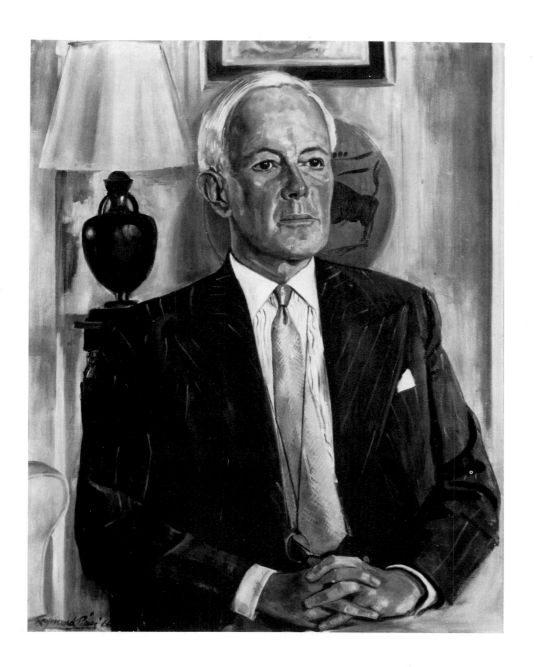

59

Avicenna c. 980–1037

Avicenna was a Persian and, it seems, an infant prodigy. He turned to the study of medicine at 16. He served various rulers and his life was hazardous. Promoted to the position of Vizier, or chief minister, by one ruler who was grateful to him for curing him of colic, then threatened by others jealous of his promotion, Avicenna's life was saved by a providential (or was it, after all?) second attack of colic. His life was to continue to be one of ups and downs – sometimes riding high as royal favourite, sometimes in gaol. In good times, Avicenna enjoyed wine and women.

Avicenna was a prolific writer – the most important of his writing being his *Canon of Medicine.* An Aristotelean, he tried to render medicine logical. Visitors flocked to his home at Isfahan to hear him teach. Western medicine from the 13th century to the 17th century strongly reflected his influence.

Beaten copper plaque, 18⅞ by 15¾ inches, by Ashrafzadeh, c. 1961

Head and shoulders, nearly profile to left; wrinkled forehead, aquiline nose, moustache with down-turned ends on upper lip, thick beard extending to ear; turban with end looped over his right shoulder, plain robe, hatched background; above, in Persian written in Nashki style on four lozenges, the famous verses of Avicenna:

Although my heart has travelled far and wide in this wilderness,
It has acquired not one whit of knowledge – and yet it has spent hours
A thousand eons have shone on my heart,
And in the end it has not achieved the perfection of a sunbeam.

On the lower margin is written in Nastaliq, in three lozenges: *On the occasion of the millenary.*
of the famous sage and philosopher Abu 'Ali Sina, born 370 A.M., died 428 A.M.

Signed on the plain rim of the embossed frame: *Ashraf Zadeh;* beyond, a border of formal flowers and intwined leaves; the copper is turned over a wooden stretcher; on this is written in ink: *Isfahan-persia | 9.9.1961.*

Presented by Dr. C. O. Minasian, October 1961.

Ashrafzadeh's portrait is of the same type as one by A. Sadighi, reproduced by Dr. Major, and which appears to be both modern and idealised. There are, of course, no contemporary portraits of Avicenna though imaginary ones were current in the West by the sixteenth century: a full frontal type appeared on the title-page of Avicenna's *Liber Canoni*, Venice, 1527. A similar portrait, shewing Avicenna in a turban surmounted with a circlet, and holding an open book was engraved in the seventeenth century by G. P. Busch as 'ex codice antiquo Galeni'. A portrait also occurs on the painted frieze in the Bodleian library, whose scheme has now been attributed to the first Librarian, Thomas James, *c.* 1616.

The donor states that the artist is the foremost brass worker in Isfahan, and has recently revived the ancient craft of manual embossing, in which the metal is worked from both front and back.

Ref: Driver, 1952, p. 12; 'Urguza "Cantica" d'Avicenne traduction par Henri Jahier et A. Noureddine' in *Histoire de la Médicine*, 1952, Mai pp. 61–71; J. N. L. Myers, 'Thomas James and the Painted Frieze', in *Bodleian Library Record*, IV, 1953, pp. 30–31; R. H. Major, *A History of Medicine*, I, 1954, p. 237; letter from the donor, 15 September 1961; *Annals*, 26 October 1961, p. 110j; the translation was kindly supplied by Dr. J. A. Boyle of Manchester University.

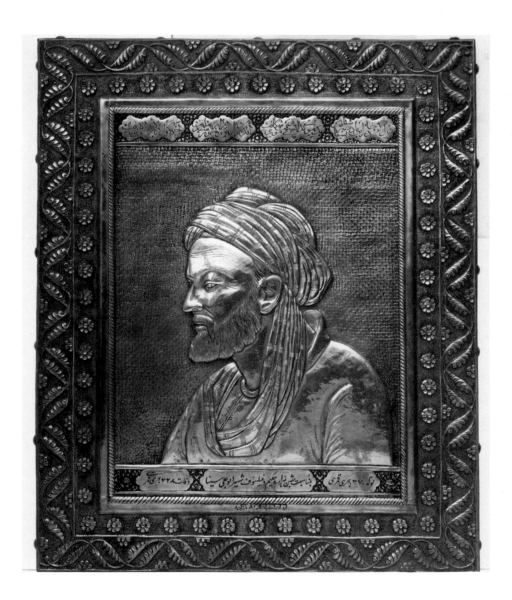

Elizabeth Margaret Baillie 1794–1876 and William Hunter Baillie 1797–1894

Children of Matthew Baillie.

Elizabeth Margaret Baillie was born in 1794. She married a Captain R. Milligan of Ryde in 1816, and died in the Isle of Wight in 1876.

William Hunter Baillie was born 15 September 1797. He seems to have been a country squire all his life. Reactionary – he closed the village reading room because he disapproved of the 'liberal literature' to be found there – and of narrow, evangelical views. When in 1851 he edited the comedies written by his aunt, Joanna Baillie, he expurgated all the oaths, commenting 'they are unsuitable to a later age'.

He married Henrietta Duff *c.* 1835, after a 'whirlwind courtship' and had eight children. He served as a Trustee of the Hunterian Collection for 25 years, and lived to a great age, dying in his sleep 23 December 1894.

Elizabeth Margaret Baillie and William Hunter Baillie

Oils on canvas, 49 ¼ by 39 ½ inches, attributed to J. J. Halls, 1802

Both whole length in the grounds of a house, partly seen in trees on left; William stands with his left arm round his seated sister's neck, she holds his left hand; he has full straight dark brown hair, parted in the centre, blue eyes, rosy cheeks, half-sleeved brown suit with white edging and buttoned waist, black shoes; she has similar but black hair, brown eyes, white half-sleeved frock, a large coral necklace and red shoes; to the left, water, with trees behind; on the right a wood with autumn foliage in foreground, a cloudy sky above their heads.

Presented by their descendant, Miss Angela Oliver, 1972.

(cont.)

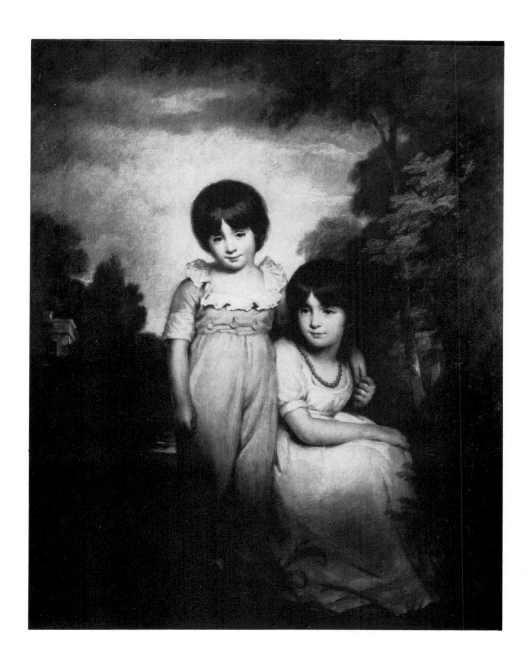

63

Miss Oliver has also presented the following portraits and miniatures: Henrietta Baillie, James Baillie, Joanna Baillie, Matthew Baillie (5) and (6), Sophia Baillie, William Hunter Baillie, John Baron, Elizabeth Denman, Thomas Denman, George III, William Hunter (4) and (5), David Pitcairn (2).

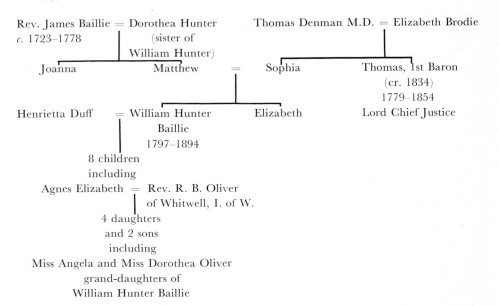

On the costume and the apparent age of the children, evidently painted just after *c.* 1800; it is a competent and attractive work. An attribution to Hoppner is traditional, but not entirely convincing; the treatment of the heads and the eyes is a little sentimental for him. The only recorded portrait, probably of these sitters is by J. J. Halls, Royal Academy 1802 (16) 'Master and Miss Baillie'. It is not impossible that this may be our picture. He was a prolific, but now rather forgotten painter, exhibiting many times at the Royal Academy 1791–1827. The only example of his work at present recorded in the files of the National Portrait Gallery library, his engraved head and shoulders of Viscount Valentia (also succeeded as 2nd Earl of Mount Norris 1816) and presumably Royal Academy 1809 (22), is insufficiently close to clinch an attribution. Comparison with Halls's portrait of the children's uncle, Lord Denman, *c.* 1819 Royal Academy 1819 (454), in the National Portrait Gallery, is also inconclusive.

Ref: A. Graves, *The Royal Academy of Arts* (S.R. and Kingsmead Reprints Ltd.), II, 1970, pp. 360–61.

William Hunter Baillie

Miniature, watercolours on ivory, 4 ¼ by 3 ½ inches, by an unknown artist

Short half length, looking right, shoulders fronting spectator; dark brown hair parted on left, curling over his right brow and covering ear tips, long brown eyebrows, pale grey-blue eyes, long nose, full lower lip; tall white collar, white shirt with small ruby(?) stud, brown waistcoat, black velvet double-breasted coat; background brown with touches of green and blue.

Presented by Miss Angela Oliver, 1972.

Although the colours are faded a little, this miniature is obviously the work of a competent professional hand, *c.* 1830 though its author has yet to be identified. Newton exhibited a miniature of 'W. Baillie, Esq.' at the Royal Academy 1824 (592), but if it was of this sitter, it is unlikely to be our miniature, which does not look like his work. Chantrey's fine marble bust of Baillie, incised and dated 1823, is in the Royal College of Surgeons of England.

Ref: R.A. catalogue 1824; W. LeFanu, 1960, p. 5 (12); M. Whinney, *Sculpture in Britain, 1530–1830*, 1964, pl. 191A; *Annals*, 27 April 1972, p. 90a.

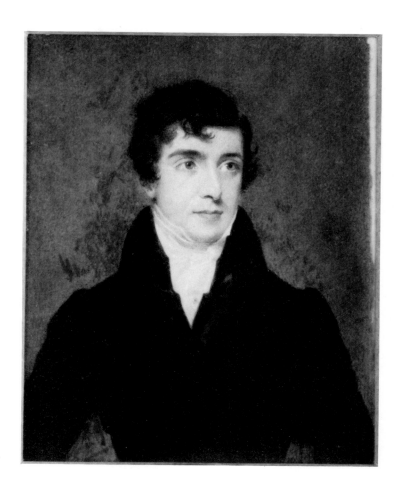

Henrietta Baillie (née Duff) ?–1856

Wife of William Hunter Baillie, whom she married *c.* 1835 after a 'whirlwind courtship'. The daughter of a Scottish minister. She is described as having been a 'great personality, handsome,' tall and 'always well dressed'. Had 8 children. Died *c.* 1856.

Oils on canvas, 36 by 29 inches, by Margaret Carpenter, 1845(?)

Three-quarter length seated to left, her right hand on red leather-bound book, left arm on chair; smooth black hair parted in centre, large dark brown eyes, lips parted; white lace head-piece decorated with flowers, black velvet frock with white lace edging and cuffs, light blue silk scarf over her left elbow, a brooch with the letter 'E' beneath a crown worn at her bosom, jewelled rings on the fourth and fifth fingers of her left hand; carved chair with red plush upholstery and arm-bands; brown background; lit from right; signed and dated, above her right hand: *Margaret Carpenter | Pinxit 1845* (?) On the bottom bar of the stretcher the remains of a manuscript label: *Henrietta Baillie (née Du[ff]) Wife | of William Hunter Baillie | by Mrs. Carpenter.*

Presented by Miss Angela Oliver, 1972.

There are two entries of £26.5s. 'Mrs. Baillie', in 1844 and 1845, in the list of the artist's work copied in 1899 from the original then in the possession of her son, Edward Carpenter. It is not clear whether they are half payments or are for two portraits: fifty guineas would be a not unreasonable price for our portrait; no replica is known. There are also two entries of £84 under the name 'Mr. Baillie' in 1839 and 1841, conceivably for her husband, but these have not been connected with any extant portrait.

Ref: 'List of Pictures and Drawings by Margaret Carpenter ... 1812 to 1864' *c.* 1899, ms in N.P.G. library.

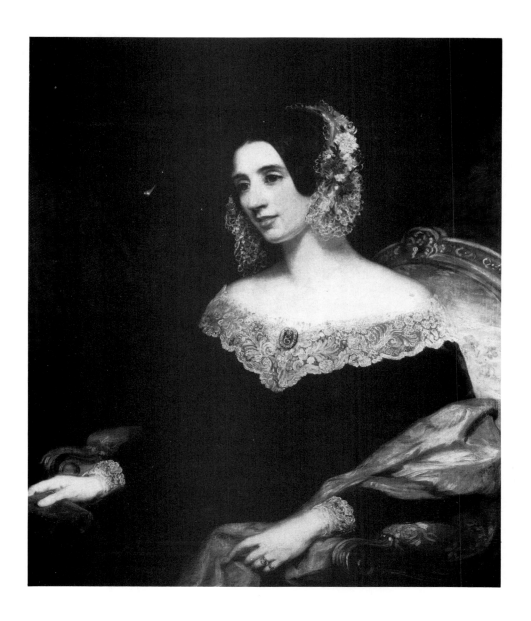

James Baillie c. 1723–1778

The Rev. James Baillie, of Hamilton and Bothwell, Lanarkshire, married Dorothea, sister of William and John Hunter, in 1758, when she was already 37. He became Professor of Divinity in the University of Glasgow in 1775. He is described as a dour Presbyterian, without much in the way of social graces, whose sermons laboured on for three hours. Nevertheless, the Baillie-Hunter marriage produced the three talented and attractive children, Agnes, Matthew and Joanna. After James's death in 1778, Dorothea returned to London and kept house for her brother William, who treated Matthew as his own son.

Oils on canvas, 29 by 24 inches, after a portrait by Robert Edge Pine of before 1777

Short half length seated, head turned back towards spectator, body to right; grey hair or wig, nearly covering ears, grey eyebrows, pale blue eyes, upturned nose, receding chin, thick jowl; white bands, black gown; plain brown background, corner of chair seen bottom left. On the bottom bar of the stretcher is written: *Portrait of Revd James Baillie | Professor of Divinity Glasgow College | Father of Mr Baillie M D Joanna and* (Agnes?) *Baillie.*

Presented by Miss Angela Oliver, 1972.

The portrait seems to be an early nineteenth century copy rather than a replica. The original and the companion portrait of Mrs. James Baillie, the latter probably commissioned by William Hunter, were painted a few years before 1777, when according to a letter to Hunter in the Royal College of Surgeons of England, Pine cut them down to their present oval size of 27 by 22 inches. This is probably the only known type. An enamel miniature 'James Baillie for Doctor Wanostrocht' is recorded but no further details are given. It is not clear whether this sitter is our James; the recipient may be Nicolas Wanostrocht, 1745–1812, a teacher of French who settled in Great Britain *c.* 1780, and worked in a school near Camberwell.

Ref: A Catalogue ... of Paintings, Drawings and Engravings by & after William Grimaldi (1751–1830), 1873, p. 37 no. 408; The Hunterian Collection ... lent by the University Of Glasgow, Iveagh Bequest, Kenwood 1952, pp. 16–17 (exhibition catalogue); *Annals,* 27 July 1972, p. 156a.

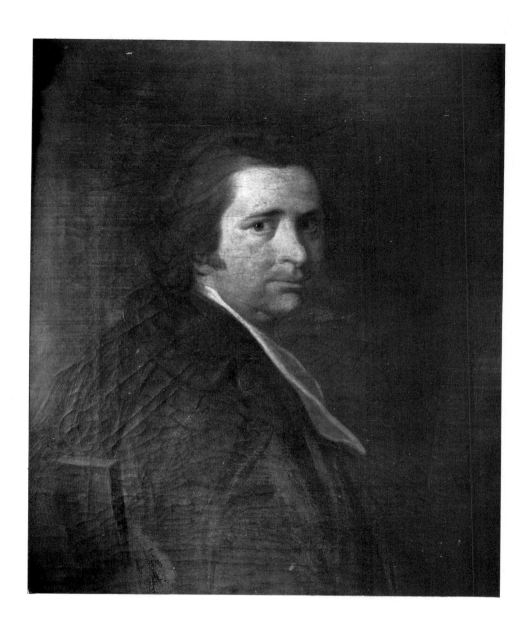

Joanna Baillie 1762–1851

Niece of William and John Hunter, and sister of Matthew Baillie. Born in Lanarkshire, a daughter of the minister of Bothwell. She was a natural tomboy and 'sat a horse as if it were a bit of herself' but life in the manse was repressive – all display of emotion was discouraged – and this may explain much of her later work as a dramatist.

When her brother, Matthew Baillie, inherited his uncle William's London house, Joanna and her mother and sister joined him there, and it was after this move that Joanna began to make her mark as a poet and playwright. Her plays generally dealt with a single emotion and lacked plot or incident, so were hardly practical for the stage. But seven of them were performed, and one of them, '*De Montfort*', with Mrs Siddons and John Kemble in the cast, ran for eleven nights. Her works, both poetry and plays, were published anonymously and their style made people of the day think that they had been written by a man – some even thought by Sir Walter Scott himself.

At their home in Hampstead, the Baillie sisters entertained many friends. One of Joanna's closest was Sir Walter Scott, who called her 'the immortal Joanna', and described her as 'the best British dramatist since the day of Shakespeare and Massinger'. Wordsworth referred to her as 'the most perfect example of a British gentle-woman'. She knew Byron well but wrote with disgust of *Childe Harold*, that 'he has shown only great want of taste (not to say the worse of it) in threading his pearls together with such a filthy string'.

She is described as a very natural, unaffected sort of person, with a pleasant personality. She nursed her mother devotedly in her last illness and lived very happily with her sister Agnes for some 45 years. She died peacefully aged 88 at Hampstead, where in the Parish Church there is a tablet and a portrait to her memory.

Miniature, watercolours on ivory, 4¾ by 3⅝ inches, by J. C. D. Engleheart

To waist, seated to left; black hair parted in centre, pale blue eyes, clear complexion; white turban with band under chin, white collar with pleated edge, purple dress with high waist, red drapery over her right forearm and behind back; settee covered in yellow material; greenish-blue curtain background, fluted column on left, a pillar on right.

Presented by Miss Angela Oliver, 1972.

The former attribution to Sir William Newton perhaps arose because of the similarity between our miniature and the small unfinished watercolour in the British Museum, engraved by H. Robinson for Joanna Baillie's *Works* 1851, and reproduced by Caw. On grounds of style it is almost certainly by J. C. D. Engleheart. This hitherto unrecorded work is the third published portrait. An oil by J. J. Masquerier was engraved by Robinson for Chambers' *Dictionary*, when in the collection of W. H. Baillie. Two miniatures, 'Miss Joanna Baillie in character', and 'with others in play', were however noted by L. G. Holland of the National Portrait Gallery *c.* 1891–2 (with a very slight sketch). S. C. Hall, *Memories of Great Men*, 1825–6, comments 'Her face was long, narrow, dark and solemn' and Sara Coleridge, *Letters*, 1834, refers to her exquisite taste in dress.

Ref: R. Chambers, *Biographical Dictionary of Eminent Scotsmen*, V, 1855, p. 22a; M. E. Wotton, *Word Portraits of Famous Writers*, 1887, pp. 13–14; L. G. Holland, *Sketchbooks*, VII, f. 48, ms. in N.P.G. library; J. L. Caw, *Scottish Portraits*, II, 1903, p. 125 pl. cviii; *Annals*, 27 April 1972, p. 90a.

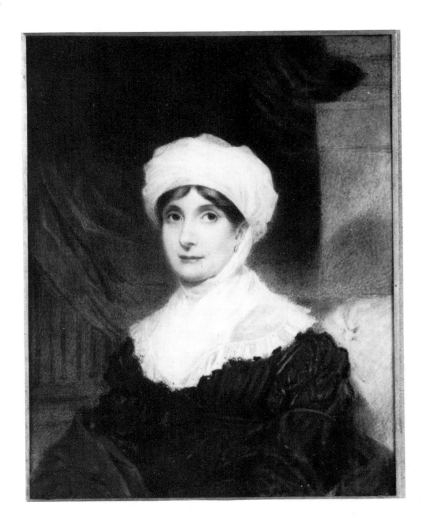

Matthew Baillie 1761–1823 F. 1790

Nephew of William and John Hunter, a kindly and highly successful practitioner; he refused a baronetcy after attending George III in his final illness.

(Catalogue I, pp. 40–45)

4. Oils on canvas, 28 by 24 inches, by an unidentified artist

Short half length to right; auburn hair brushed back, dark brown eyebrows, dark blue eyes, long nose, prominent lower lip; white shirt and cravat tied in bow, yellow waistcoat with orange stripe, dark blue double-breasted coat; red curtain drawn back revealing landscape on right; inscribed, on the curtain *M | Baillie | M.D.*, and, illegibly, on the rolled paper in his right hand. On the sealing paper at the back of the picture is written: *Matthew Baillie b 1761 d 1823 MD Oxford* author of *Morbid Anatomy of the Human Body;* the back of the canvas is stamped *281 | 17 | 70 MATLEY | — ACID.*

Source and date of acquisition unknown.

This unrecorded portrait may be amateur work; the costume and apparent age suggest it was painted within a few years of 1800.

Ref: Catalogue, I, 1964, pp. 40–45.

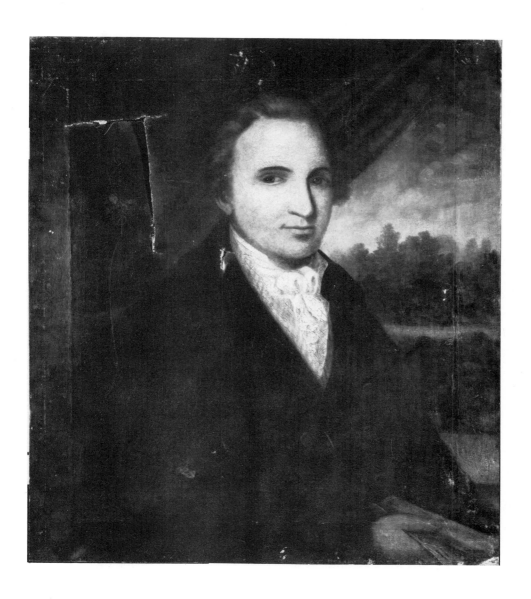

Matthew Baillie]

5. Miniature, enamel, 4¾ by 3¾ inches (sight), by Henry Bone, 1810, after the portrait by John Hoppner

Half length, seated to right, hands not seen; short grey hair, brushed back, reaching to collar, long dark brown eyebrows, pale brown eyes, tip of nose curving slightly down, receding chin, fresh complexion; grey velvet double-breasted coat partly unbuttoned, white collar and cravat; green upholstered chair; red curtain background; lit from top left. Inscribed at the bottom of the slip *ENAMEL H BONE*, the *H B* in monogram; an old ink label on the backing board reads: *Matthew Baillie M.D. | Born October 27th 1761 | Paid for the Enamel 45. guineas | Frame 7 guineas |* , in another hand, *Henry Bone | 15 Berners Street | London |* , and yet another, *From a Picture of Hoppner's.*

Presented by Miss Angela Oliver, 1972.

Copied from the Hoppner engraved in 1809, which was presented to the College in 1895; Bone's reduced, squared drawing in the N.P.G. is inscribed: '*Dr Baillie after Hoppner | for Mrs. B. Jan 7 1810*'.

Ref: Henry Bone, *Sketchbooks*, III, f. 13, N.P.G. library; *Catalogue*, I, 1964, no. 1, pp. 40–42; *Annals*, 27 April 1972, p. 90a.

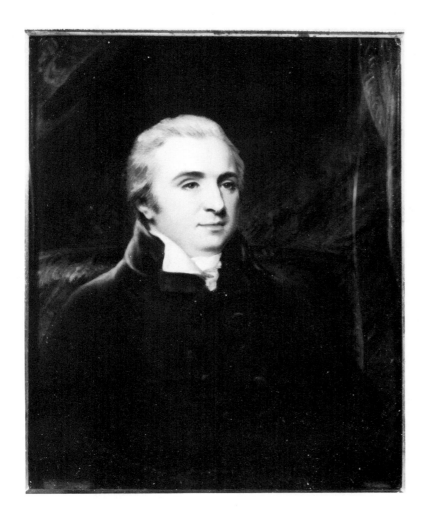

Matthew Baillie]

6. Oils on canvas, 30¼ by 25 inches, attributed to Thomas Barber, c. 1806

Short half length to right, hands not shewn; short grey hair covering ears, dark brown eyes, dark grey eyebrows, straight nose, double chin; white cravat, double-breasted green coat; green(?) background. On the back of the canvas a stamp: *755 17 75.*

Presented by Miss Angela Oliver, 1972.

Quite near the portrait in the College painted by Lawrence in 1806, but slightly different in pose and by a less able hand. It is tempting to propose his pupil Thomas Barber, of Nottingham, whose work it rather resembles; no portrait of Matthew Baillie by him is recorded, but he painted other members of the family.

76   *Ref: Catalogue,* I, 1964, pp. 42–44; *Annals,* 27 July 1972, p. 156a.

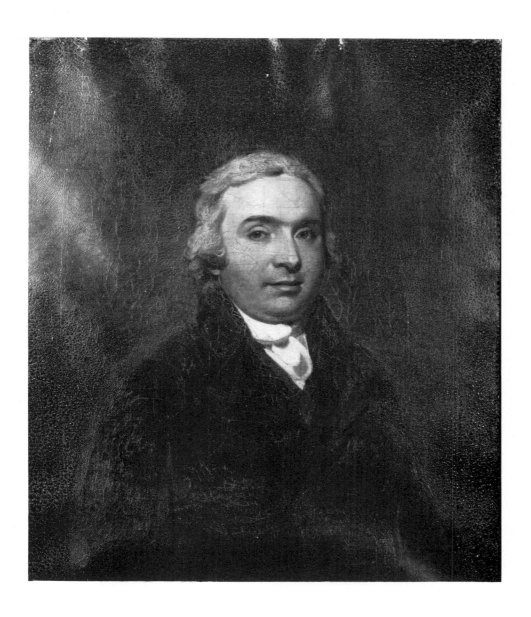

Sophia Baillie 1771–1845

Daughter of Dr Thomas Denman, physician accoucheur, of London. She married Matthew Baillie in 1791 and her husband claimed that in all their years together they never exchanged an unkind word. On Matthew Baillie's death, his wife gave the College the gold-headed cane which had belonged to Drs Radcliffe, Mead, Askew, William and David Pitcairn and her husband, and also the painting by Zoffany of William Hunter and members of the Royal Academy (see Cat. I, p. 233).

Oils on canvas, 29¾ by 24¾ inches, attributed to Thomas Barber

Half length seated to left, her right hand resting on left wrist; full black hair dressed high parted in centre and tied with band, grey eyebrows, pale blue eyes, straight nose, lips closed; cross-over black quarter-sleeve dress with gold armbands, white blouse open at neck, underneath red cloak with white lining; she is silhouetted against a greenish-blue sky, shading to orange bottom left; there are pentimenti in her left arm, the elbow being originally nearer the picture edge; remains of manuscript label on the back in the same hand as on the portrait of Henrietta Baillie: [w]*ife of Mathew* / [si]*ster of the first* / [rest illegible].

Presented by Miss Angela Oliver, 1972.

As Mr. R. E. Hutchison kindly suggests, the portrait is close to the work of Thomas Barber, whose portrait of her brother, the judge, Thomas, 1st Baron Denman, is in the Castle Museum, Nottingham.

Ref: *Annals,* 27 July 1972, p. 156a; information R. E. Hutchison, Esq., Scottish National
78 Portrait Gallery.

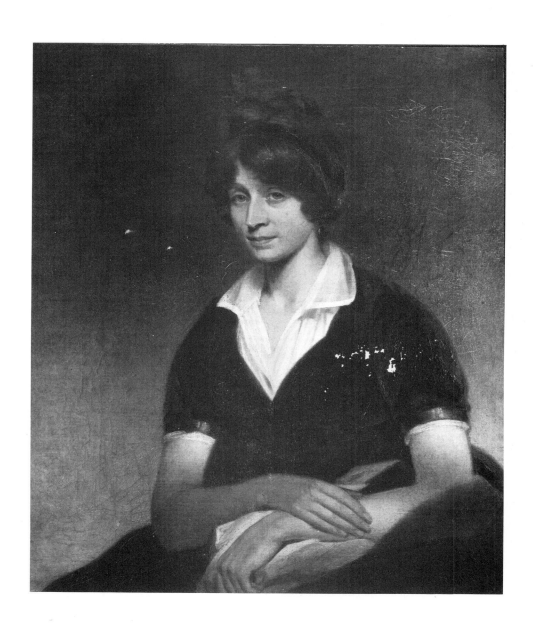

John Baron 1786–1851

Friend of Edward Jenner and Matthew Baillie – and biographer of the former. Born in St. Andrews; he studied medicine at Edinburgh, then practised in Gloucester until poor health forced him to retire in 1832. 'Creeping palsy' disabled him physically, but his mind remained unaffected. He upheld the theory that tubercles were hydatids become solid (a respectable theory at the time, in which John Baron was by no means alone) and, although the theory was later discredited, it helped him – together, no doubt, with such friends as Baillie and Jenner behind him – to win admission to the Royal Society. He gained a better reputation as a writer than as a scientist.

Baron advocated more humane treatment of the mentally ill, and was a founder of the Medical Benevolent Fund.

Oils on canvas, 30 by 25 inches, by Henry Room, c. 1838

Short half length to left, head turned back towards right; receding curly white hair reaching to ear, grey eyebrows, grey-brown eyes, straight nose, thick lower lip; tall white collar, bottle green cravat, matching waistcoat, white shirt, darker brownish-green coat with black velvet collar; background of grey sky, lighter brown on left.

Presented by Miss Angela Oliver, 1972.

The type was engraved by W. Holl. The impression on the engraving in the N.P.G. is dated 1847, but is possibly a reissue, as according to Burgess (179) the engraving was for Pettigrew's *Medical Portrait Gallery*, 1838–40. Our oil is the only known type and the only recorded version, apart from the engraving and may well have belonged to Matthew Baillie, who was a friend of the sitter.

Ref: Dictionary of National Biography, III, 1885, p. 269; *Annals*, 27 July 1972, p. 156a; Burgess, 1973, p. 23.

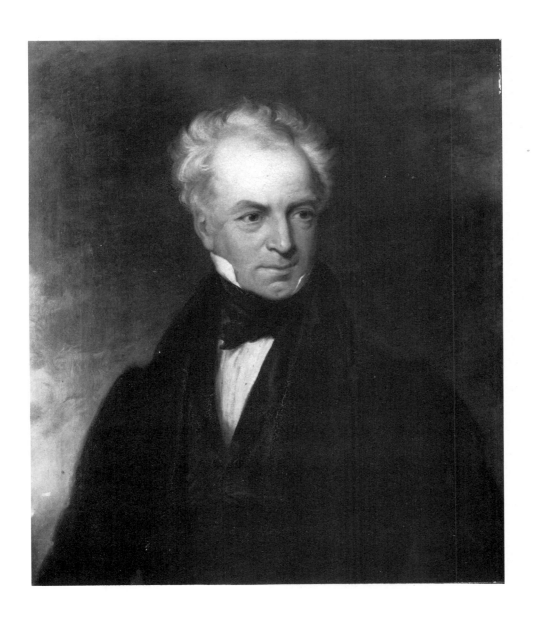

William Battie 1704–1776 F. 1738 P. 1764

Son of the Rev. Edward Battie of Modbury, Devon, formerly an assistant master at Eton. Born in Devon and educated at Eton and King's College, Cambridge.

Battie wanted originally to be a lawyer but was forced by unknown circumstances to turn to medicine. His lectures on anatomy at Cambridge were attended by, among others, Horace Walpole.

He was already successful in practice at Uxbridge when he inherited a handsome sum from a relative. He moved to London in 1737, where in time he became physician to St Luke's Hospital for Lunatics, which he had been instrumental in founding and which opened in 1751, and he also became proprietor of a large private asylum. In 1742 Battie was elected a governor of Bethlem Hospital (for a fee of £50) and in 1754 he took over another 'madhouse', in Clerkenwell Close. He retired from practice when made President of the RCP: the first 'psychiatrist' – and only one? – to be so. Died from the effects of a stroke 1776, extremely rich. Horace Walpole estimated his estate at *c.* £100,000.

Spoken of by friends as a 'funster', he was regarded as an eccentric – e.g. he sometimes dressed like a labourer – and was often satirized: e.g.

First Battus came, deep read in worldly art,

Whose tongue ne'er knew the secrets of his heart,

In mischief mighty, tho' but mean of size,

And, like the Tempter, ever in disguise.

See him, with aspect grave and gentle tread,

By slow degrees approach the sickly bed;

Then at his Club behold him alter'd soon –

The solemn doctor turns a low Buffoon ...

Battie – the expression 'batty' does not, alas, derive from William Battie – helped to make the treatment of insanity respectable. He was the first teacher of the subject in England, if not in the world, and wrote a *Treatise on Madness*, which challenged some of the traditional thinking on the subject. He saw that madness was not a single illness, requiring a single form of treatment, and was the first 'mad doctor' to treat his patients as individual cases. He observed that some patients recovered spontaneously and that some actually recovered when the (very harsh) treatment of the day was stopped. And he divided madness into two basic categories: 'original' and 'consequential'.

82

[William Battie

William Battie]

Oils on canvas, 43½ by 35½ inches, by an unknown artist

Nearly whole length seated, looking round to right, a pamphlet in his right hand, his left hand on arm of chair; grey wig touching shoulders, grey eyebrows, blue eyes, long nose, double chin, white neckband, grey-green coat with gold buttons and long button holes, matching waistcoat with gold edging, dark breeches, white wrist ruffles; bookshelves on left, plain brown background; the pamphlet inscribed, beneath an elevation of St. Luke's Hospital: *REASONS | For the ESTABLISHING and Further | ENCOURAGEMENT | OF | St. Luke's HOSPITAL | FOR LUNATICKS. | TOGETHER | With the RULES and ORDERS | FOR THE | GOVERMENT thereof.* Inscribed top right: *Doctor William Battie, 1704–1776. Physician Kings Scholar, Eton. Kings College | Cambridge 1722. Founded Battie Scholar- | ship at Cambridge 1747. Fellow of College of | Physicians 1738. Censor 1743, 1747, 1749. | President 1764. Physician to St. Luke's | Hospital:* the pamphlet has a blue paper cover, and the left hand side of the title-page is dark, as if it had been folded down the middle. The words *for the* have been brought up by the painter into the previous line and put into lower case otherwise the inscription follows the title page of the pamphlet in the Royal College of Physicians library.

Purchased from Sotheby's, 1 August 1973, lot 163, anonymous property; anonymous property, Robinson and Fishers, 19 February 1925, lot 47, as by W. Hoare, bought for the Wellcome collection; subsequently with D. Minlore.

The inscription, not visible in a photograph in the National Portrait Gallery files taken in 1939, is possibly an addition by D. Minlore. The correspondence between the lettering bottom left and the title-page of Battie's pamphlet has aroused some misgivings: only paint sampling and analysis would perhaps indicate whether the paint here is contemporary, retouched in part or modern. But even if the last were the case, the provenance of the picture is strongly in favour of its authenticity, since it can be seen in a photograph of the dining room of Prideaux House, the daughter-in-law's family home, before the sale in 1924.

Ref: Correspondence with Sir Harry Rashleigh, Bt., 15 October 1973; unpublished information L. M. Payne, Esq.

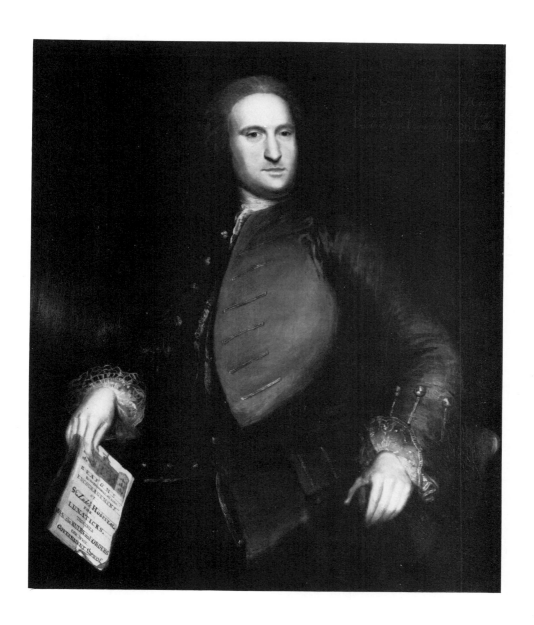

Sir Harold Esmond Arnison Boldero 1889–1960
F. 1933

Born August 22 1889, the son of John Boldero JP; educated at Charterhouse, Trinity College, Oxford, and Middlesex Hospital Medical School. He served in France during World War I as a regimental medical officer and then as D.A.D.M.S., and was twice mentioned in despatches. He returned to the Middlesex in 1919 with the rank of major. There, he became well known as an outstanding teacher, and his special interest was in paediatrics. He got on exceptionally well with children and with their parents. With Lord Webb-Johnson, he was to be responsible for the idea of the Courtauld research wards where patients were cared for jointly by a member of the Hospital staff and a professor from one of the School's basic sciences.

In 1934, Boldero was appointed Dean of the Middlesex Hospital Medical School, a post which he held for 20 years. It was a traumatic period, which he negotiated with great skill, including as it did the 2nd World War (and all the upheaval that meant) and its aftermath. As an undergraduate dean, he was made in 1939 a sector officer in the Emergency Medical Service and helped organize the air-raid casualty services. At the same time, he made sure that the School's teaching continued without interruption.

He gained the reputation of a great administrator and in 1941 became Treasurer of the RCP. In 1942, he was appointed Registrar and was to be one of the College's great Registrars, serving in this capacity for 18 years, under the three Presidencies of Moran, Brain and Platt. He dedicated himself no less to the College than to the Middlesex. He was in the thick of the National Health Service negotiations when Lord Moran was President. He was knighted in 1950.

In his youth, Boldero had been athletic and good enough to play as centre-half in the English hockey team. Manner austere, distant, reserved; a witty man on social occasions, sometimes caustically so; given to understatement; kind; perhaps shy; believed in orthodox procedure. A dedicated and respected committee man, it was felt that his administrative duties took preference over his development as a teacher and clinician.

Oils on canvas, 30 by 25 inches, by Joyce Aris, after a portrait by Harold Knight of c. 1957

Short half length to right; smooth receding grey hair, dark brown at sides, grey eyes, dark brown spectacles, straight nose; white collar, plain grey tie, scarlet gown over dark brown coat and waistcoat; quill, standish and book on table on right.

Commissioned by the College, and painted between July and October 1963.

The original, which was exhibited at the Royal Academy 1957, was commissioned by the

Medical School Council of the Middlesex Hospital in November 1956; sittings began December 1956 and the picture was delivered after the close of the Royal Academy summer exhibition 1957. A photograph of the sitter was taken for the National Photographic Record in 1940.

Ref: R.A. catalogue 1957 (306); als from Joyce Aris 31 July, 31 October 1963, from Prof. A. Kekwick to Dr. R. Bomford, 13 October 1967.

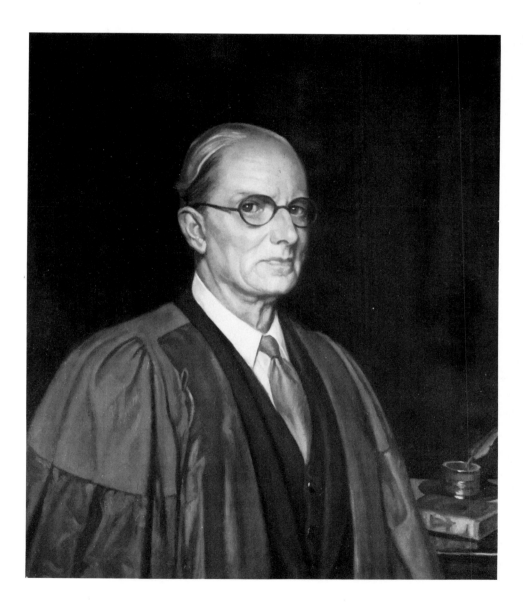

Edward Browne 1644–1708   F. 1675
P. 1704–1708

Edward Browne was the eldest son of Sir Thomas Browne, author of '*Religio Medici*', and was born in Norwich. He qualified as bachelor of medicine at Trinity College, Cambridge, and travelled abroad the next year to Paris and Italy, in the company of Sir Christopher Wren and others. In 1667 he obtained his MD at Merton College, Oxford. The same year he was made a Fellow of the Royal Society, and in the following year set out on another journey, farther afield this time, returning in 1669. Three years later he married the daughter of Dr Christopher Terne, a Fellow of the Royal College of Physicians, and in 1673 he published an account of his travels in East Europe, remarkable for the scrupulous accuracy of its reporting. Browne never tried to embroider his experiences – an unusual quality in those days – and his contemporary, Dr Johnson found the book dull and made no bones about it, but Charles II, to whom Browne was a physician-in-ordinary, spoke of him as 'learned as anyone at the College, and as well-bred as any at court'. Other written works of his included translations of the lives of Themistocles and Sertorius for an edition of Plutarch's *Lives*.

Edward Browne's patients included the celebrated Earl of Rochester, and it was through his friendship with the Marquis of Dorchester that the latter promised his library to the College on his death.

Oils on panel, 13⅛ by 10¾ inches, by an unknown artist

Half length to right, his right elbow resting on ledge, left hand not shown; mid-brown hair, thin light brown curving eyebrows, dark blue eyes, long upper lip with faint moustache, blue jowl, cleft chin, middle-aged appearance; broad white cravat with lace edge, white shirt with matching lace front and cuff, half-sleeved black coat; plain dark brown background, a mountain with twin summit seen through an opening on the right, inscribed at bottom: *M : OL;* a small white object held between the thumb and forefinger of his right hand, a blue stone beneath the opening on the right. Inscribed on the back: *Sir Thomas Brown | of Norwich M.D.*

Purchased from Sir Solly Zuckerman (Lord Zuckerman) January 1969. From Bryan Hall, Banningham, near Aylsham, Norfolk (bt. G. Hayes, Swaffham); from the collection of David Stewart 11th Earl of Buchan, 1742–1829.

Although not closely dateable, the costume suggests the first decade of the Restoration, and the sitter's age, not perhaps quite as young as at first sight, nevertheless rules out the elder and more famous Browne. In view of the inscription and the chalk figure *16* still visible on the back, this must be the picture from the 15th Earl of Buchan's collection sold by Dowells, Edinburgh, 22 January 1944, lot 16, as Sir Thomas Browne. A panel of almost the same size, lot 6, was sold as Edward Browne, but described as resting his right hand on a bust. This may have been the portrait from which an engraving was published by Harding in 1801 after an original in Buchan's collection. Buchan was a sometimes indiscriminate collector; it is not known when the portrait came to him. The engraving, which might not represent the whole picture however, shows a younger man in a different cravat and clothing, including drapery over the sitter's left shoulder, and a jerkin sewn together down the front opening. The object held in the right hand in our portrait is now nearly indecipherable, but might be a white stone mineral specimen, such as is mentioned in Browne's *Travels*. He visited Olympus which he there described as a mountain with several summits. The iconography of Edward Browne is overshadowed by and confused with that of his father, but it seems improbable that he would have sat, at any rate frequently, and no further portraits are recorded.

Ref: E. Browne, *A Brief Account of Some Travels in divers Parts of Europe ... With some Observations on the Gold, Silver, Copper* etc. ..., 1685, p. 35 and passim; F. Johnson, *Catalogue of Engraved Norfolk and Norwich Portraits*, 1911, p. 27; Burgess, 1973, p. 53.

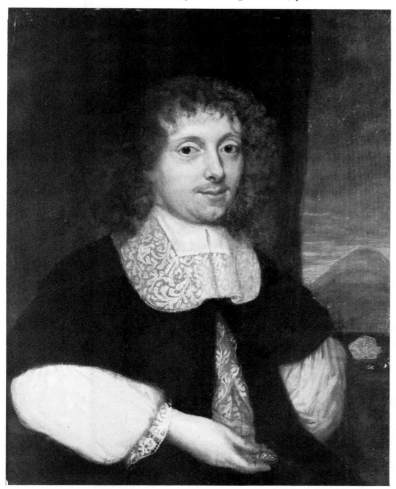

John Conolly 1794–1866 F. 1844

This proves to be a pastiche of Lawrence's portrait of Durham, 1st Earl of (q.v.)

Sir John Conybeare 1888–1967 F. 1926

Known as 'Cony' to his colleagues, Sir John's life was bound up with Guy's Hospital in one way or another.

Born in Oxford, and educated at Rugby; New College, Oxford; Guy's Hospital. Read classics at Oxford before reading medicine. Fought in World War I while still a medical student, completed his studies, returned to battle and gained the Military Cross.

1929 saw the publication of *Textbook of Medicine*, edited and partly written by him. Cony favoured plain, clear speech and writing.

Warden of Guy's College in 1923 for 14 years. In 1946, he was elected a governor, though he did not actually retire from the staff until 1953.

A great champion of causes; very popular; sociable – entertained a good deal and belonged to many dining clubs; manner said to have been 'brusque and forthright', but essentially courteous; a bachelor, he always had two or three students sharing his flat and felt he had many sons; he played golf with Lord Nuffield and it was probably through this association that Guy's was to benefit so much from Lord Nuffield's generosity.

Oils on canvas, 30 by 25 inches, by (Alfred) Neville Lewis, c. 1950

Half length to left, head looking back towards spectator and cigarette in his right hand which rests on back of chair, left hand on lapel of coat; straight grey hair thinning on top, bushy black eyebrows, mid-brown eyes, long nose, cleanshaven tanned complexion; soft light blue shirt, dark blue tie with thin light blue and red diagonal stripes (R.A.F.), plain light grey coat and trousers; dark blue background; lit from left. Signed in red, top right: *Neville Lewis*. An undated label of the Royal Society of Portrait Painters on the back of the frame, with the address: *Neville Lewis, c/o TLT Lewis FRCS, Guys Hospital*.

Presented by the Trustees and Executors of the sitter, January 1970.

The only version, commissioned by the sitter; exhibited at the Royal Society of Portrait Painters in 1950 (98).

Ref: R.S.P.P. catalogue 1950, p. 14; als. from executors, G. H. Greenwell and W. N. Mann 22 February 1967, and from Mr. T. L. T. Lewis, 18 March 1976.

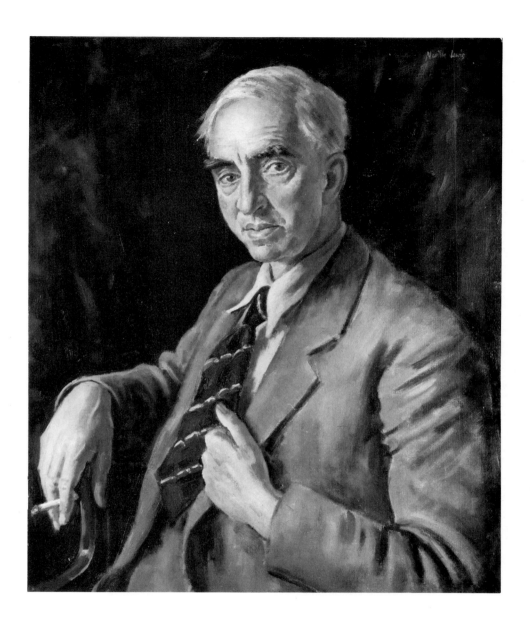

91

Thomas Forrest Cotton 1884–1965 F. 1931

A Canadian, Thomas Cotton was born in Quebec 4 November 1884, and educated in Montreal. He qualified in medicine at McGill University. In 1913 he moved to London and worked under Sir Thomas Lewis. Then back to Montreal for a time to run a department of electrocardiography. The Military Hospital, Hampstead, had been established for research into the heart disorders of soldiers and it was here that Thomas Cotton resumed work in London in 1914. He collaborated with Osler and other pioneers in the heart world to investigate 'soldiers' heart' or effort syndrome, as Sir Thomas Lewis named it.

He was the first to recognize clubbed fingers as a sign of subacute bacterial endocarditis and probably his most important original contribution was a report to the Medical Research Council on this condition.

In 1924 he was appointed to the National Hospital for Diseases of the Heart and, because of his long experience in the subject, was invited to act as consultant cardiologist to Queen Alexandra's Military Hospital and the Ministry of Pensions.

A good mixer, he communicated cheerfulness and optimism to patients and staff. Successful investments in Canada enabled him to make a major bequest towards the Osler Room at the College, so named at his request. His ashes lie next to Osler's in the Osler Library at McGill.

Oils on canvas, 22 by 18 inches, by David Jagger, c. 1926

Head and shoulders, slightly to left; smooth light brown hair, pale grey eyebrows, pale blue eyes, full lips; white collar with green stripe, black tie, black coat, red handkerchief, plain green waistcoat; plain black background, lit from left; signed, bottom right, *JAGGER*.

Received with Dr. Cotton's bequest to the College and hung, 1967.

92   *Ref:* al. from Mrs. M. A. Cotton, 17 October 1967.

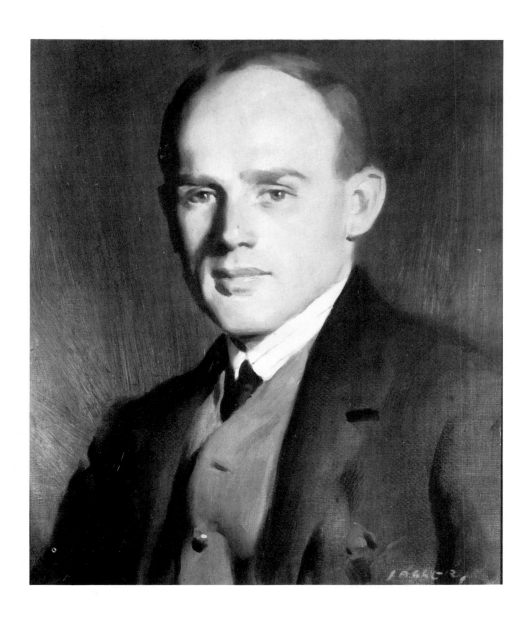

93

James Curry d. 1819 L. 1801

James Curry was born in Antrim, N. Ireland, but it is not known precisely when. In 1784 he graduated MD from Edinburgh and, hoping to practise his craft in Bengal, got himself hired as surgeon to a native of that country. But his health forced him to return to England and for some years he was physician to Northampton County Hospital.

His next move was to London, where he worked as physician to Guy's. He helped to popularize the use of mercury in the treatment of patients and one of his written works bears the title '*Examination of the Prejudices commonly entertained against Mercury, as beneficially applicable to the greater number of Liver Complaints, and to various other forms of Disease, as well as to Syphilis*'.

About James Curry the private man, nothing appears to be known.

Miniature, watercolours on ivory, 2 5/16 by 2 13/16 inches, oval, by an unknown artist

Head and shoulders to left; high greyish-white hair surmounted by two curls, pale brown eyebrows, grey eyes, full bottom lip, firm jaw; he wears steel spectacles, white neckband and shirt, black coat with a high collar; blue background. A modern inscription on the back: *Dr James Currie | Physician to Guy's Hospital | 1802–1819 | from the Collection of Mrs Dont* (?) | *the actor*, and, in another hand, *& later, the property of | Sir John Conybeare KBE MC FRCP.*

From the collection of Sir John Conybeare, presented by his executors, October 1968.

Mrs Dont (?) is very uncertain, and has not been identified. The artist is competent, but there seems little prospect of identifying him, or her. The fashion and hair style of the portrait indicate a date of *c.* 1805. A portrait by F. Simonau was engraved by I. Mills in 1819.

Ref: O'Donoghue, I, 1908, p. 543; al. from the executors, G. H. Greenwell and W. N. Mann 22 February 1968.

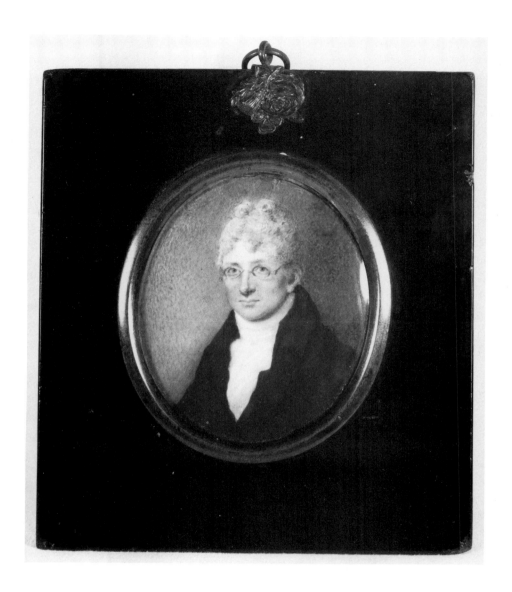

Elizabeth Denman (Wife of Thomas Denman) 1747–1833

The daughter of Alexander Brodie, an army accoutrement maker of Queen Street, Golden Square, London, and aunt of Sir Benjamin Brodie, Elizabeth was described as 'a handsome and engaging young gentlewoman of Scottish descent.'

In 1770 she married Thomas Denman (q.v.) who later wrote '... it would have been impossible to have chosen a wife more suitable to my disposition and circumstances. Her manner was amiable, her disposition gentle, her understanding naturally good ... She is frugal without meanness, temperate and cheerful and it is impossible for any two people to have lived together with more harmony ...'

Thomas and Elizabeth Denman had three children, Margaret who married Sir Richard Croft, Sophia (q.v.) who married Matthew Baillie, and Thomas who became Lord Denman. The last named was born in Queen Street, Golden Square, now Denman Street, named after him.

Elizabeth may have been gentle and engaging; she was also a woman of strong character: '... she drew up forty-six rules for the regulation of her own conduct in the minutiae of daily life, e.g. the precise extent to which she was to indulge in dinner parties and morning visiting.'

Miniature, watercolours on ivory, 3 ¼ by 2 9/16 inches, by George Engleheart

Short half length to right, head turned back towards spectator; wispy black hair, black eyebrows, blue eyes, large nose, thin lips; pale blue bonnet with double lace foreedge and large bow on top, pale blue lace collar and plain black cross-over dress with broad black lace edge; grey background, lighter on right; lit from left. Inscribed in ink on the backing paper of the frame: *This portrait of my mother, | kindly lent to me by my | nephew William Hunter Baillie | March 23, 1845. | must be restored to him at | my death D.*

Presented by Miss Angela Oliver, 1972.

Formerly known as Sophia Baillie, 1771–1895, on apparent age and date the sitter is far more likely to be of the previous generation. The inscription is presumably in the hand of Thomas, 1st Baron Denman (cr. 1834), William Hunter Baillie's uncle. On the strength of this our miniature should represent Elizabeth, née Brodie (*d.* 19 January 1833) who married Thomas Denman M.D., 1 November 1770, rather than her daughter, Sophia, William Hunter Baillie's mother. No portraits of Elizabeth are available for comparison, though a marble bust by C. Moore of a Mrs. Thomas Denman, exhibited at the Royal Academy 1828, presumably was of her. If Baillie is really the sitter's name, Mrs. James Baillie (1721–1806) might be indicated, but there is little resemblance to the Pine of her in the Hunterian (above, under James Baillie). There is on the other hand, a good deal of similarity between the features in our miniature, especially the nose, and the oil of Sophia. Hitherto unattributed, the miniature is a typical and fine George Engleheart. Although possibly incomplete, the published list of his sitters 1775–1813 does not include any Baillies or Denmans and the likelihood is that the miniature was painted between 1813 and the artist's death in 1829; but the costume suggests a date near the beginning of this period.

Ref: R.A. catalogue 1828 (1146); G. C. Williamson and H. L. D. Engleheart, *George Engleheart*, 1902; *Annals*, 27 April 1972, p. 90a.

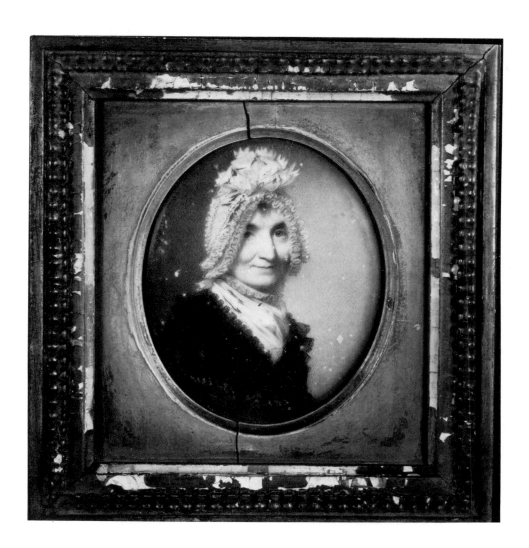

Thomas Denman 1733–1815

Born at Bakewell, Derbyshire, the son of an apothecary, Denman began his medical studies at St George's Hospital, but then entered the medical service of the Navy, first as surgeon's mate, then as surgeon. After nearly ten years he left the Navy and had the good fortune to come under the influence of William Smellie, turning his main interests towards midwifery.

After graduating MD at Aberdeen, he practised in Winchester to such poor effect that even the Navy seemed preferable. Failing to re-enter the service, he had the luck to be granted £70 a year for occasional duties on a royal yacht. With an easier mind he began to give lectures on midwifery, so successfully that he was appointed physician accoucheur to the Middlesex Hospital from 1769 until 1783, by which time his popularity in private practice overwhelmed his hospital duties.

Denman seems to have gone through life with a direct simplicity, regular habits, and a care for the common man, which he may well have owed to his naval up-bringing.

He and his wife Elizabeth (q.v.) had three children. The son, Thomas, became Chief Justice of England, and of the twin daughters, one married Matthew Baillie and the other Sir Richard Croft MD.

He was buried in St James's, Piccadilly, where there is a simple tablet to his memory.

Oils on canvas, 30 by 25 inches, by an unknown artist

Half length seated to left, head tilted to left, eyes directed at spectator, a red book in his left hand; receding straight white hair, pale blue eyes, prominent nose, narrow lips, double chin, fresh complexion; white collar, brown double-breasted coat buttoned up with black velvet collar, matching waistcoat; red upholstered bench, dark brown background.

Presented by Miss Angela Oliver, 1972.

Although this portrait has been known as William Denman, 1821–1907, it bears considerable resemblance to the portrait of Thomas Denman, engraved by W. Skelton after L. F. Abbott in 1792 presumably after the original lent by his son Lord Chief Justice Denman (Thomas, 1st Baron Denman, 1779–1854) to the third National Portrait Exhibition, South Kensington, 1868 (34). The hair is straighter in our portrait, but it might well represent Thomas Denman about 1810. Apart from the Abbott, the only portraits recorded, other than engravings, were a miniature by M. Haughton R.A. 1810 (625) and a drawing by J. J. Halls R.A. 1812 (782). An anonymous engraving after T. C. Lochée, 1788, might indicate a medallion, since Lochée sometimes worked for Wedgwood; a small engraving was also published as the frontispiece to Denman's *Aphorisms on the ... Use of Forceps*, etc., 1824.

Ref: O'Donoghue, II, 1910, p. 33, VI, 1925, p. 127; exhibitions cited in text; *Annals*, 27 July 1972, p. 156a.

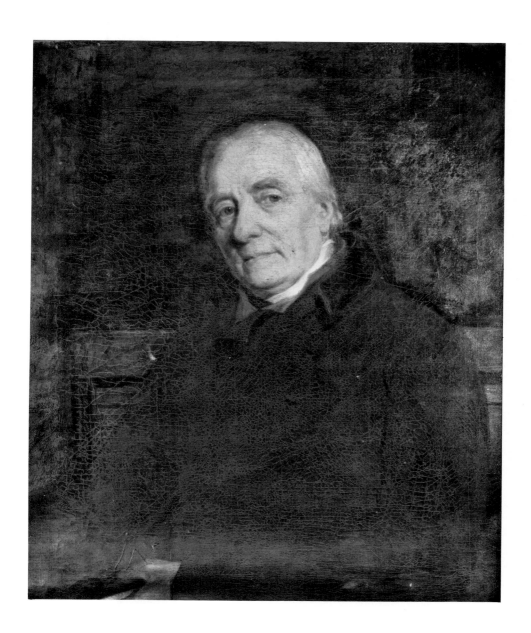

Sir Charles Dodds Bt. 1899–1973
F. 1933 P. 1962–66

Educated at Harrow County School and Middlesex Hospital Medical School he remained throughout his working life a 'Middlesex man'.

At only 25, he was appointed Courtauld Professor of Biochemistry at the Middlesex and, in 1928, he became the first Director of the Courtauld Institute of Biochemistry until his retirement from both the Chair and the Directorship in 1965. He radically reorganized the teaching of biochemistry and chemistry there, insisting that they be integrated. As a 'chief', he was a sympathetic listener to the problems of his staff and allowed them considerable autonomy.

In 1942, he was elected FRS, and in 1954 knighted for the synthesis of various new oestrogens – notably stilboestrol, which he had discovered in 1938 and which, amongst its other uses, had been employed in the control of carcinoma of the prostate – and for his Directorship of the Courtauld Institute of Biochemistry.

The first 'laboratory man' to be elected President of the RCP; although not a practising physician, his contributions to medicine were substantial. His Presidency has been described as 'unobtrusive and efficient'. He was an excellent Chairman, limiting his own words to the fewest possible, and discouraging others from wasting time.

During his Presidency, he frequently expressed concern about the possible effects on women of oral contraceptives taken over many years, and presided over a committee set up by the Medical Research Council to look into the matter.

He was doggedly loyal to his staff who in turn were devoted to him. A faithful member of the Society of Apothecaries, he found in it what others gained from their universities: a love of ceremony and tradition and fine wine and companionship; unusually, he was Master for two successive years, and his influence on the wine cellar lasted at least a generation.

Despite the comfort of his family – his son married the daughter of Sir Daniel Davies, FRCP – he survived with difficulty the death of a beloved wife.

Oils on canvas, 35⅞ by 28 inches, by Raymond Piper, 1967

Half length seated to left, leaning on his left elbow and holding formula for stilboestrol in his lap; grey hair brushed down, bald on top, horn-rimmed spectacles, pale blue eyes, short nose, lips parted, double chin, a pimple or spot below his left ear, fresh complexion; soft white collar, red silk tie, mid-grey pin stripe suit, the jacket open; gold watch with metal strap, chair back upholstered in grey; plain green background, lit from left. Signed and dated, bottom left, in black: *Raymond Piper 1967*.

Commissioned by the College; received 1967.

A photograph was taken in 1970 for the National Photographic Record.

Ref: Annals, 26 October 1967, p. 148a.

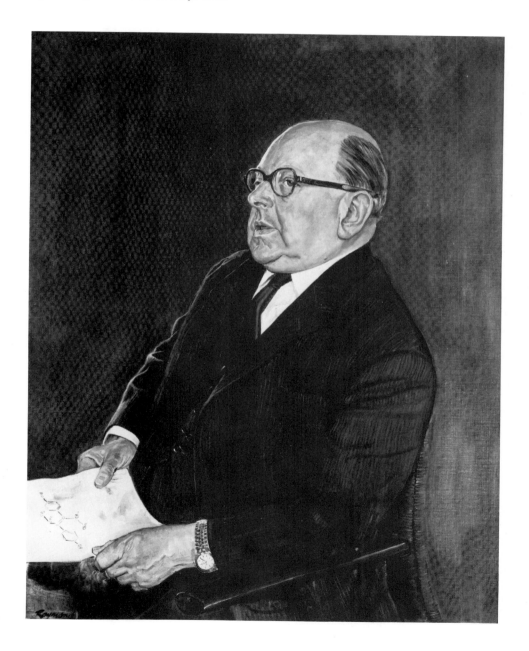

John George Lambton,
1st Earl of Durham 1792–1840

Whig politician and a fire-eating radical. He pushed for electoral reform and finally helped to prepare the first Reform Bill (not as reformed as he would have liked it to be). Hated political dealing and conciliation and was always quarrelling with someone – once fought a duel with one of his critics.

Married twice and, through his second wife became son-in-law of Earl Grey, in whose administration he served. He apparently was the stronger personality of the two men; at any rate, he had considerable influence with his father-in-law. But Melbourne, when approached, refused to make room in his cabinet for Lambton because of the latter's overbearing temper and lack of tact.

In 1838 Lambton was appointed High Commissioner of Lower Canada and Governor-General of the British provinces of North America but resigned in the same year when criticized for his high-handed actions by the British Government, which withdrew its support from him.

Het tried once for the leadership of the Party but failed. Without doubt, a very able man: energetic, ambitious; but uncomfortable as a colleague because of his arrogance and unwillingness to compromise. He had many of the qualities that were the downfall of Coriolanus.

He died quite young, only 48 years old, at Cowes. It is said that his health had never been good.

Oils on paper(?) laid down on canvas, 11⅜ by 9⅜ inches, by an unknown artist

Half length, holding glass and bottle, body to left, head slightly to right; curly black hair, black eyebrows, brown eyes; brown coat, red drapery over; in an interior, a cupboard right with jars and small skeleton on top. Inscribed on the backing canvas: *John Connolly* (sic) *F R C S* etc., three lines now illegible.

The attribution of Conolly (he was F.R.C.P.) to the Surgeons and the letters '-ence', presumably for Lawrence, then legible in the inscription, raised doubts about the authenticity of the portrait which proves to be a pastiche of Lawrence's portrait of the first Earl of Durham, probably painted over the engraving of it by J. Cochran.

102   *Ref:* O'Donoghue, II, 1910, p. 107.

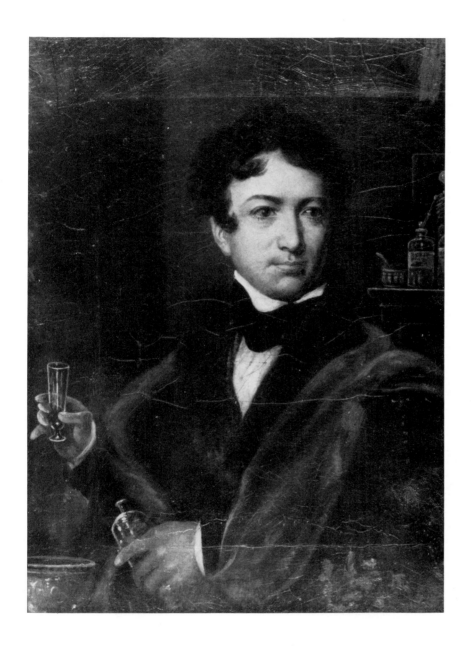

103

Horace Evans, 1st Baron Evans of Merthyr Tydfil
1903–1963 F. 1938

A Welshman, born on New Year's day, the son of an organist and conductor. The father must have hoped his son would grow up to be a musician like himself, for when Horace was 12 he was sent to the Guildhall School of Music. However, Horace reverted to his grandfather's interest in medicine (he had been a pharmacist) and at the age of 18 entered the London Hospital Medical School. Apparently he was regarded as only an average student, giving no hint then of the great physician he was to become.

Work at the London Hospital with Arthur Ellis and Clifford Wilson on hypertension and nephritis secured his appointment as assistant physician in 1933 and physician in 1947.

In 1944 Evans was appointed physician to Queen Mary and this was the beginning of an association with the royal family that only ended with his death; in 1949 physician to George VI; 1952 physician to Elizabeth II. Created Baron in 1957.

At the College, he was examiner, councillor, Censor and Senior Censor and it was he who persuaded the Wolfson Foundation to contribute splendidly towards the College's new building in Regent's Park.

Evans disliked committee work and professional politics. A man of great charm, he enjoyed dining out and was an enthusiastic attender at the dinners of the Society of Apothecaries, of which he was Senior Warden when he died.

He was beloved for his unfailing kindness; never in the least pompous or unapproachable; the nurses at the London referred to him affectionately as Horace; apart from delighting in his friendships and good food, he also loved horse-racing, though he did not gamble; his manner was relaxed and serene – he never appeared to be in a hurry despite the demands on his time; he was throughout his life an unassuming man, and a good listener, waiting patiently for everyone else to speak before giving his own quietly delivered opinion; devoted to his patients, he worked long hours and took an interest in their personal problems as well as in their physical condition. Many of his patients were doctors and their relatives.

In his private life he bore with quiet courage the death of a daughter and serious illnesses of his wife, and remained gentle, courteous and considerate throughout the very painful illness leading to his death at the age of 60.

Oils on canvas, 39⅞ by 29⅞ inches, by Joyce Aris after Sir James Gunn (Herbert James Gunn)

Three-quarter length seated to front, his right hand on crossed knee, his left arm on mahogany chair; smooth receding black hair, blue eyes, transparent spectacles, long lips, fleshy chin; black tie, white collar and shirt, plain slate-grey double-breasted suit, gold cuff links; grey drapery behind, lit from left. Painted on Herga canvas supplied by Windsor and Newton.

Commissioned by the College, 1966.

Copied from the original in the Clinical Theatre West, London Hospital. A good likeness, it received the warm approval of the sitter's daughter. Photographs were taken for the National Photographic Record in 1962 and 1969.

Ref: Annals, 28 July 1966, p. 217; *Commentary*, July 1968, p. 82.

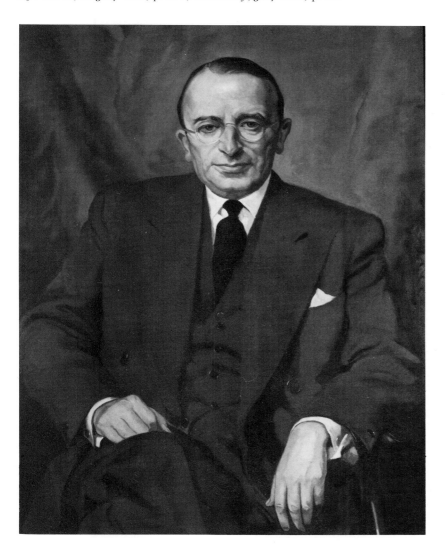

Sir John Forbes 1787–1861 F. 1844

Born at Cuttlebrae, Banffshire, John Forbes was educated at Fordyce Academy, where he formed a lifelong friendship with Andrew Clark, and Aberdeen Grammar School. From there he went to Marischal College and thence to Edinburgh University for a year. Having taken the diploma of surgery in 1807, he joined the Navy as an assistant surgeon until 1816. He returned to Edinburgh to graduate in 1817 and, for the next five years, practised general medicine in Penzance. In 1822 he moved to Chichester, where he was largely responsible for the foundation of the local infirmary. He was a popular physician and the practice was a lucrative one, but it was through his written works that he became famous. In 1821 his translation of Laennec's *Treatise on the Diseases of the Chest* helped to establish auscultation in England His next task in 1832–35 was the joint editorship with Alexander Tweedie and John Conolly of the *Cyclopaedia of Practical Medicine*.

In 1840 he moved to London in order to be conveniently situated for the editing of the successful and highly regarded *British and Foreign Medical Review*, which he had initiated in 1836. The move meant a financial sacrifice despite his appointment that year as physician to the Queen's Household. Ironically, it was an article by Forbes himself that contributed to the decline of the *Review*. Entitled *Homoeopathy, Allopathy and 'Young Physic'*, the controversial article was thought by many of his colleagues to be too sympathetic to homoeopathy. Forbes continued to receive many honours, however, and in 1853 was knighted by the Queen.

In later years he took up such varied subjects as phrenology, clairvoyance and mesmerism, giving free range to the curiosity that appears to have motivated him throughout his life.

Oils on canvas, 29⅛ by 37¾ inches, by John Partridge, c. 1847

Half length to right, reading, the fingers of his right hand in pages of a book held in the left; short receding grey hair, dark eyes, side whiskers, white shirt, dark coat; on a table in the right foreground, paper, a small red leather case, and quill(?) and ink; the rest of the picture is obscure, being extensively damaged by the artists' use of bitumen. On the back an excise mark TB 2 47 and a colourman's stamp *BROWN | 163 | HIGH HOLBORN | LONDON |*. An old manuscript label, written in ink *Sir John Forbes MD FRS DCL etc | This Picture painted by Partridge was given to John De Burgh Forbes | by his Godfather John Forbes Clark Esqr | the 3rd of May 1861 | Picture painted about 1847.*

The date and source of acquisition of the picture is not known; but Partridge's notebook suggests a version was painted for the sitter.

The notebook, a transcript of which is in the library of the National Portrait Gallery, records in 1848 'John Forbes Esqr M.D. 52. 10' and in 1851 '– Forbes Esqre 52. 10'. He had already in 1844 listed 'Master John Forbes' at '78. 15' and in 1845 there is an entry 'Mrs George Forbes 63. 0.' '52. 10' would be appropriate to the size of our canvas. The two entries

106

rather suggest two portraits, but if '– Forbes' was also our sitter, only the portrait in the College is known. A three-quarter portrait by T. H. Maguire 1848 was engraved in lithograph. Partridge's portrait was engraved by W. Walker, as a private plate in 1852. A painting stated to represent the sitter in early life is in the Board Room of the Royal West Sussex Hospital, Chichester.

Ref: *Illustrated London News*, xxxix, 1861, p. 390; John Partridge, notebook, ms. in N.P.G. library; O'Donoghue, II, 1910, p. 234; F. W. Steer, *The Royal West Sussex Hospital* (The Chichester Papers No. 15), 1960, pl. 3.

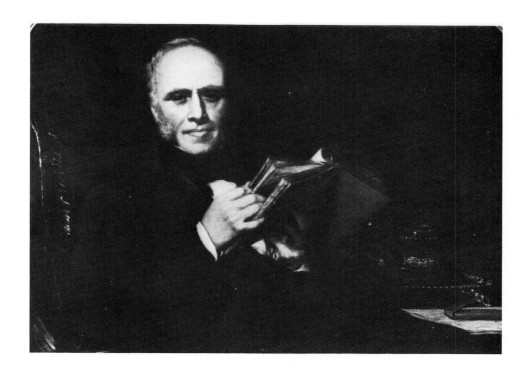

John Freind 1675–1728 F. 1716

Classicist and chemist, specialist in fevers and politician. Committed once to the Tower and released when Richard Mead refused otherwise to treat the Prime Minister, Robert Walpole. Became physician to George II and Queen Caroline.

(Catalogue I, pp. 170–173)

2. Medallion, boxwood, 7 by 5 inches, oval, by an unknown artist

Head and shoulders, slightly to right, short curly ('classicised') hair, protruding lower lip, double chin; toga with brooch on his right shoulder.

Source and date of acquisition unknown.

On the backing board, now incomplete, an old inscription in ink: *Dr. John Friend* (sic). / *born 1675. Died 172*[8] / *buried in Westmin*[er] / *Abbey*. Also the remains of two seals: at the top in green and on the bottom in red wax; the green wax has the initials [G?]*WD* in the centre within an oval lettered —— *MED*.

(See also Medals pp. 204–205.)

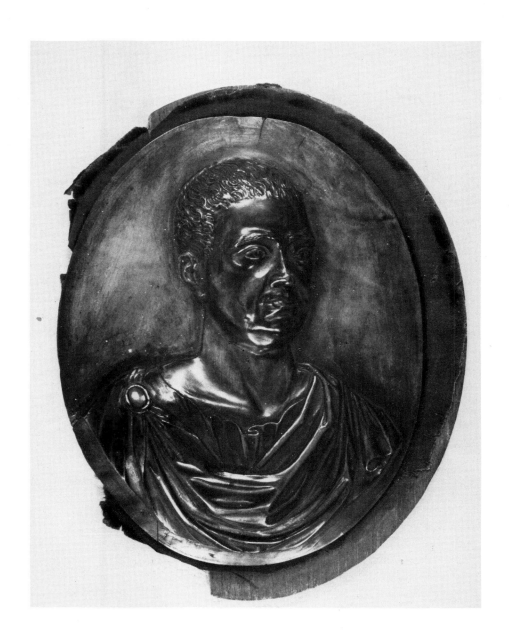

John Farquhar Fulton 1899–1960 F. 1953

Born in St Paul, Minnesota, son of a physician and ophthalmic surgeon and related to Robert Fulton, pioneer of the steamboat, John left school at 16 and worked with a surveying team on the West Coast. He enrolled at the University of Minnesota in 1917. He failed his entrance examination to Harvard because he had discovered writers such as Tolstoy and had neglected his studies for his new love, but then enlisted in the Army and entered Harvard as a 'veteran'. Graduated *magna cum laude*, and was admitted as a Rhodes Scholar to Magdalen College, Oxford, in 1921.

Seconded to Cambridge to help Sir Arthur Shipley in the preparation of his classic work, *Life*, on elementary biology – the book is dedicated to Fulton. Under Sir Arthur's influence, he became a gastronome and his hospitality later was famous.

While University demonstrator in Physiology at Oxford, he was the pupil of Sir Charles Sherrington. He published papers in *Journal of Physiology* and *Proceedings of the Royal Society*, and with Dr W. Francis (Osler's nephew) and Mr Reginald Hill of the Bodleian Library, compiled the *Bibliotheca Osleriana*, and was at this time inspired with the desire to collect medical books. He left Oxford, after graduating D. Phil. in 1925, and returned to Harvard. It was as assistant neurological surgeon at the Peter Bent Brigham Hospital that he came under the supervision of Harvey Cushing, whose biographer he would eventually be – indeed, this biography, published in 1946, has been compared with Cushing's own biography of Osler.

In 1928 he went back to Oxford to be a Fellow at Magdalen, but in 1930 was in America again, having been given the Chair of Physiology at Yale, later to be known as the Sterling Professorship. He called his department 'the Laboratory' and it was here that his work on the brain of the chimpanzee enabled Egas Moniz to perform the first prefrontal lobotomy on man in 1936. Work done on the physiology of man at high altitudes was to be of particular value to the British and American Air Forces in the Second World War. In 1938, his classic textbook, *Physiology of the Nervous System*, was published.

On Cushing's death in 1939, Fulton helped to establish the Cushing Library at Yale, something that Cushing had dreamed of, and out of this sprang a new university department. In 1951 Fulton was appointed Sterling Professor of the History of Medicine and soon made Yale the mecca of all medical historians.

A handsome man in his youth, and a humanist; John Fulton never actually met the man who had so much influenced his life – Osler – because he arrived at Oxford two years after Osler's death, but he knew Lady Osler well and became steeped in the Osler tradition.

He died suddenly on 29 May 1960 in Connecticut, aged 60.

[John Farquhar Fulton

John Farquhar Fulton]

Oils on canvas, 35⅛ by 28⅛ inches, by Deane Keller 1965, after a portrait by Sir Gerald (Festus) Kelly c. 1957

Half length, seated in a library and looking across table, spectacles in his right hand, a handkerchief in his left; close cut wavy grey hair, parted in centre, arched grey eyebrows, pale blue eyes, long thin upper lip; soft white collar held with gold tie-pin, blue tie, light grey jacket with red rosette in button hole (Legion of Honour), white handkerchief in breast pocket, matching grey waistcoat, watch with steel strap, tortoiseshell spectacles; on the table an open quarto, and an engraving unfolded, and an octavo, both bound in calf; in the foreground a tray in which the top paper is addressed, upside down to the viewer, *Deane Keller | Yale Art Gallery | ... John Fulton*, and on the right of the table a blue paper slip on which is written *John Fulton | Gerald Kelly*; books behind and to left, a shuttered window top left. Inscribed in black on the back of the canvas: *Copy by Deane Keller | Yale Univ. | New Haven | Conn., U.S.A. | 22 Feb 1965 completed | from original of | Dr. John F. Fulton | by | Sir Gerald Kelly | past P.R.A.*

Given by Mrs. Lucia Fulton, July 1965, for whom it was painted by Deane Keller.

Copy of the portrait by Kelly in the Yale Medical Historical Library.

112   *Ref:* R.A. catalogue 1957 (585); *Annals*, 29 July 1965, p. 89; *Commentary*, July 1968, p. 82.

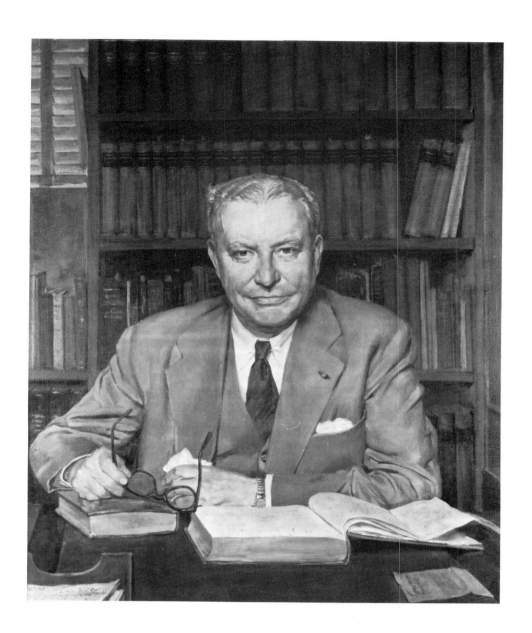

113

Sir Alfred Baring Garrod 1819–1907 F. 1856

Born in Ipswich and educated there in the Grammar School, and later at University College Hospital, London, where he won the Galen medal of the Society of Apothecaries for botany, and gold medals with his MB and MD.

In 1847, as assistant physician, he discovered the presence of uric acid in the blood of patients with gout and in 1859 published a treatise on *Gout and Rheumatic Gout* (a landmark in its own field); he also separated rheumatoid arthritis as a disease distinct from gout.

In 1851 he became full physician and Professor of Therapeutics and Clinical Medicine at University College, but left his own school in 1863 when elected physician to King's College Hospital and Professor of Materia Medica and Therapeutics at King's College.

He was knighted in 1887, and in 1890 appointed physician-extraordinary to Queen Victoria.

At the College he was censor and vice-president, and the first recipient, in 1891, of the Moxon Medal. At the time of his death he was the second oldest surviving Fellow.

One of his six children was Sir Archibald Garrod, FRCP, FRS.

Oils on canvas, 43 by 33 inches, by Sir Hubert von Herkomer, 1882

Three-quarter length seated, body slightly to left, head directed at spectator, hands on arms of leather-upholstered chair; grey hair full at sides, thinning on top, long near white side-whiskers, point of chin clean-shaven; arched grey eyebrows, bluish-grey eyes, thin gold spectacles, long lips, some red in cheeks; double-breasted black coat, black bow, white shirt, grey trousers; plain brown background; signed bottom right with initials *H H82*.

Given by Dr. John Garrod to the Heberden Society, 1974; on indefinite loan to the College.

Herkomer exhibited a portrait of Garrod at the Grosvenor Gallery in 1883, which may be the above. E. Nora Jones exhibited a miniature at the R.A. in 1893.

114   *Ref: The Grosvenor Gallery ... Summer Exhibition*, 1883 (188); R.A. catalogue 1893 (1299).

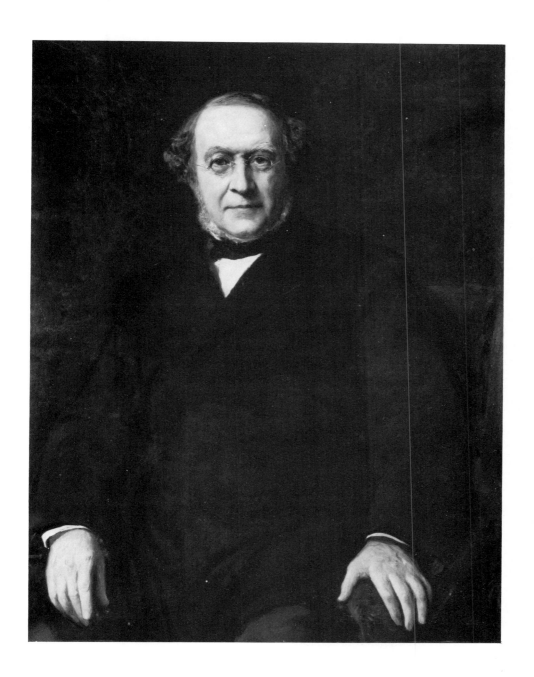

Samuel Jones Gee 1839–1911 F. 1870

A brilliant teacher, remembered through his mannerisms, at St. Bartholomew's, and first to identify coeliac disease.

(Catalogue I, pp. 178–179)

Samuel Jones Gee with his daughter Edith Thyra Gee

2. Miniatures, each watercolours on ivory, 2 ½ inches circular, by an unknown artist.

Nearly profile to left; receding white hair, grey eyebrows, blue eyes, thick white moustache with down-turned ends on upper lip, large chin; white collar, grey double-breasted suit; shaded blue background. Framed as a pair with his daughter, who is in profile to right; she has light brown hair dressed high, brown eyebrows, blue eyes, straight nose, firm chin, long neck with single string of pearls, pale mauve dress, with elaborate white collar.

Bequeathed by the sitter's daughter, October 1963.

Ref: al. from the solicitors, Baileys, Shaw and Gillett, 11 October 1963; *Catalogue* I, 1964, pp. 178–9.

116

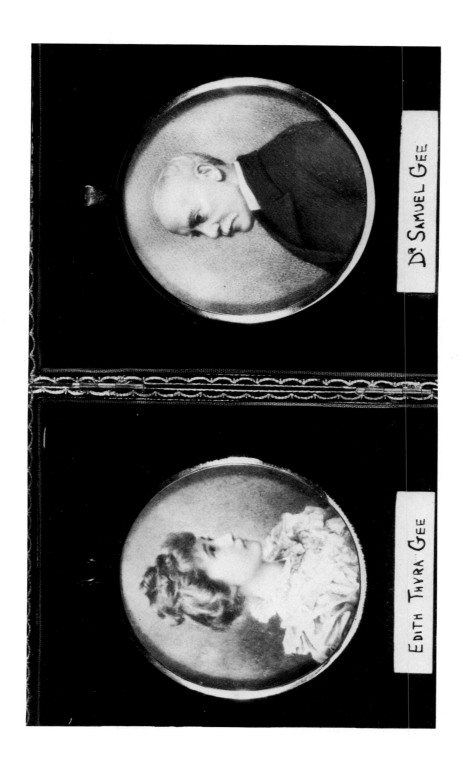

DR SAMUEL GEE

EDITH THYRA GEE

117

George III 1738–1820

'Farmer George' – as he later came to be known because of his fascination with agricultural matters – was the grandson of George II and the first of our Hanoverian kings whose mother tongue was English. He was dominated by his mother and exhorted by her to 'be king'. In an attempt to wean him away from her George II offered him £40,000 a year. His grandson took the money but stayed with his mother. He grew up believing in his own infallibility, a belief that was never shaken in spite of his disastrous relations with his ministers.

In private he was a very simple man whose lack of dignity was regarded with contempt, but now he would probably be praised for informality. He was religious, intolerant of change, pennypinching, a faithful husband, and begot in all 15 children. His court was dull.

Through the 60 years of his reign, George was persecuted and harassed in one way or another – ridiculed, stoned, and even shot at. And by 1765, a new and horrible form of persecution began. In this year George had his first attack of what for over two centuries was assumed to be madness. It was not until 1967 that Macalpine and Hunter published their diagnosis of porphyria, which has aroused wide interest. The conventional treatment for madness in those days was severe and must have added to the king's misery. His doctors were hamstrung both by ignorance and by a rigid protocol which insisted that the king always be the first to speak. By 1809, George was totally blind. He died, a pitiable old man, 11 years later, and remains for historians, and to a lesser extent for doctors, a controversial figure.

Oils on copper, 13¼ by 11 inches, oval, by an unknown artist, after a painting by Sir William Beechey of 1799/1800

Head and shoulders slightly to left, shoulders fronting spectator; grey eyes and eyebrows, lips parted, grey wig tied in queue, heavy jowl, flushed complexion; black hat with black cockade, scarlet jacket with black collar and revers, gold lace and epaulettes, star of Garter. An old manuscript label on the back nearly illegible *Picture of King George 3rd given by to Matthew Baillie MD.*

Presented by the Misses Angela and Dorothea Oliver, January 1970.

Our portrait is a reduced head and shoulders copy after the whole length portrait by Beechey at Buckingham Palace in general officer's uniform, with his charger, held by a groom, and a troop of cavalry in the distance. This was shewn at the Royal Academy in 1800, and seems to have been painted as a companion to the whole length of the Queen painted by Beechey at Windsor in 1796. The type was frequently repeated, both life size and in miniature.

Ref: O. Millar, *The Later Georgian Pictures in the collection of Her Majesty the Queen*, I, 1969, pp. 5–6, II, pls. 156–7; *Annals*, 29 January 1970, p. 204a.

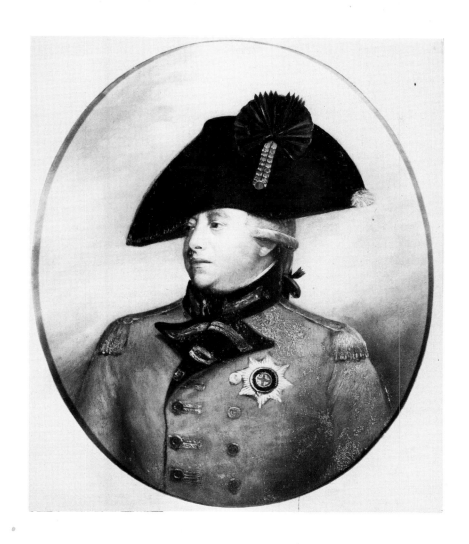

Sir George Godber 1908– F. 1947

Born in Bedford and educated at Bedford School and New College, Oxford, where he rowed for the University, George Godber qualified in medicine from the London Hospital and added shortly afterwards a diploma in public health. In 1939 he joined the staff of the Ministry of Health, and by 1960 had risen to the top as Chief Medical Officer.

During the Second World War, Godber was a Principal Regional Medical Officer for the North Midlands Region and undertook with others a survey of the region's hospitals. He served also as a member of the Working Party on Medical Staffing Structure in the Hospital Service under the then Sir Robert Platt's chairmanship. A dedicated believer in the National Health Service, he has fought courageously to defend its ideals against the opposing pressures of doctrinaire politicians, of both main parties, and of no less doctrinaire doctors.

Knighted in 1962 and advanced to GCB in 1971, Sir George retired in 1973 but continues to ride fearlessly to the crusades, in loyalty to the Health Service, and against two old public health adversaries, venereal disease and smoking. He looks to the day when society will reject promiscuity, and make smoking a socially unacceptable habit. In recognition of the value to public health of his influential leadership, he was awarded the gold medal in Therapeutics of the Society of Apothecaries in 1973, and he is an Honorary Fellow of the Royal Society of Medicine.

A quiet man – unless roused – it was characteristic of him that at his retirement party there was no smoking, no alcohol, no speeches,

Bronze bust, hollow cast, 21 ¼ inches high, by David McFall, 1974

Head and shoulders, cut off just below the breast pocket, head tilted slightly up and to right; close cut hair, parted on left, furrowed brow, a monocle in his right eye; soft shirt, collar and tie, jacket. Incised on the back, bottom left: *McFall 1974.*

Presented to the College by Fellows and Collegiate Members in recognition of Sir George's services as Chief Medical Officer from 1960 to 1973.

120   *Ref: Annals*, 25 July 1974, Doc. 17a.

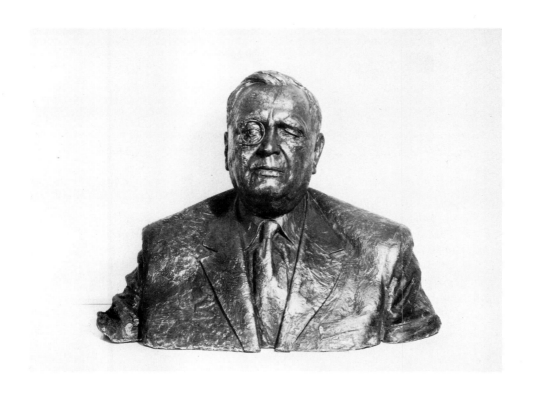

Sir Archibald Gray 1880–1967 F. 1918

Born in South Devon, and educated at Cheltenham College, University College Hospital, London, and later the University of Berne, Switzerland.

Gray set out to be a gynaecologist but UCH invited him to succeed Henry Radcliffe Crocker and he went to Berne to study dermatology. He took up the appointment on his return and was to be his generation's leading dermatologist in this country. Whatever speciality had been opened to him it is likely he would have been equally successful.

During World War I, he was attached to the general staff of the War Office and acted as consulting dermatologist in the Army Zone of the British Expeditionary Force, with the rank of lieutenant-colonel RAMC (TA). He was knighted in 1946.

From 1948 to 1962 he was adviser in dermatology to the Ministry of Health. At the College he gave the Harveian Oration in 1951, and in 1952 he was President of the first International Dermatological Congress to be held after World War II, which gave him special pleasure.

Towards the end of his long life, illness incapacitated him though his mind remained alert and vigorous. He had been an 'excellent committee man'; he was not one for the limelight, but he liked to wield behind-the-scenes influence – the politics of his profession fascinated him. Physically he was a little man. He could be irascible at times, but never bore grudges.

Sir John Gray, FRS, former Secretary of the Medical Research Council, is his son.

Oils on canvas, 30 by 25 inches, by Rodrigo Moynihan, 1956

Half length seated to left, arms by side, hands not seen; grey hair brushed flat, pale brown eyebrows, pale blue eyes, rimmed spectacles with gold frame, long thin lips, clear complexion; white collar, patterned blue tie, blue shirt, open bluish-grey coat, matching waistcoat, with chain through fourth button, his left shoulder higher than his right; mahogany chair back low on right; green background. Signed top right and dated *Moynihan '56*. There are pentimenti above the shoulders. On the back of the canvas is the stamp of the suppliers Roberson & Co. of 71 Parkway NW1.

Property of the British Association of Dermatology, who commissioned the portrait and presented it to the sitter *c.* 1958. After Sir Archibald's death, it was given to the Association by his widow in 1968, and lent by them to the College.

A photograph was taken for the National Photographic Record, 1952.

122   *Ref:* als. from E. Gray, 25 April 1968; from S. C. Gold, 10 May 1968.

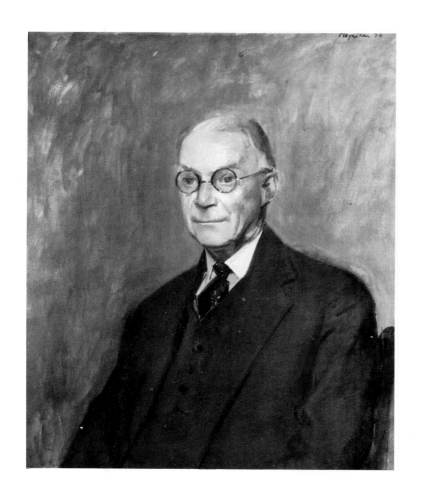

123

Baldwin Hamey Sr. 1568–1640 L. 1609/10

Descended from Odo de Hame, who was present at the siege of Acre, the father of Baldwin Hamey Jr. was born in Bruges and obtained his medical degree at Leyden. It took him a long time to graduate but when he finally did he distinguished himself, and his professors recommended him as physician to the Czar of Russia. He held this appointment for five years. In 1598 he returned to Holland, married and went to live in London.

The victim of a fever epidemic, Baldwin Hamey Sr. died in 1640, and was buried in the church of All Hallows, Barking, where there is an epitaph composed by his distinguished son. In his Will he bequeathed the sum of £20 to the College.

(Catalogue I, pp. 196–201)

Oils on canvas, 25⅜ by 20½ inches, by an unknown artist, 1633

Head and shoulders, looking at spectator; greying hair, dark brown eyebrows, dark brown eyes, white close-trimmed pointed beard and moustache with falling ends, broad face, ruddy complexion; black cap trimmed with white lace, large white ruff, plain black costume; plain brown background, lit from right; coat of arms top left. Inscribed top right: *.AETATIS.SVAE 64 | . A°. DNI. 1633* the AE in monogram; a faint inscription in black, not necessarily contemporary, to left of the sitter's head: *Bald: Hamey | Senr M.D. | Van S(?)oamer Pinx.*

Given anonymously 28 July 1967; anonymous property, Christies, 28 July 1967, lot 284; bought at a country dealer's about five years before.

No other portraits are available for comparison. Ralph Palmer, the sitter's great-grandson, and author of the manuscript biography in the College library, possessed, *c.* 1733 at his house in Little Chelsea, portraits of Hamey and his wife by Cornelius Jonson. The oil of Hamey has been equated with the signed and dated Jonson, 1624, last heard of when lent to the R.A. 1879 (77) by J. F. Stanford. Only the immediate provenance of our portrait is known; its identity rests at present on the internal evidence. The coat of arms, which appears to be contemporary or nearly so, seems correct: gules, a fesse between a roebuck, courant in chief, or and three estoiles in base argent. The rubbed inscription below gives the sitter's identity, though the attribution is unlikely; while there is a strong Netherlandish influence, the portrait is surely by a much more robust hand than Van Somer. The prominent, though perhaps slightly later, inscription top right is a year out: Hamey would have been sixty-five in 1633, but this might be due to the change in the calendar, or even to strengthening of the last figure of the date.

Ref: J. J. Keevil, *Hamey the Stranger*, 1962, p. 179, and refs. therein cited; *Annals*, 26 October 1967, p. 148a.

124

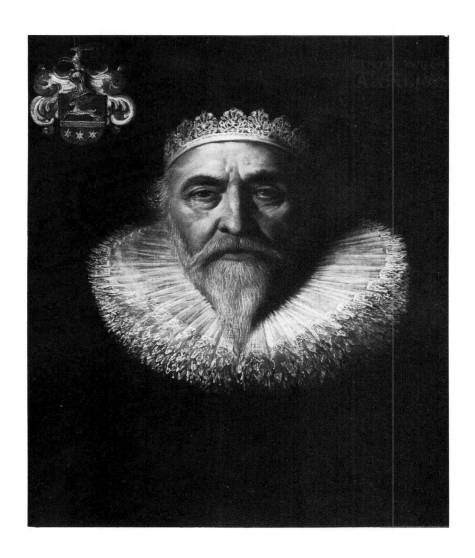

Dorothy Christian Hare 1876–1967   F. 1936

Born 14 September 1876 at Bath. She was educated privately till the age of 19 – then, Cheltenham Ladies' College; London School of Medicine for Women, graduating 1905.

House appointments at the Royal Free and Elizabeth Garrett Anderson Hospitals for 5 years.

1910–16 practised general medicine in Cambridge; 1916 Malta, attached to the RAMC.

1918–19 appointed chief medical director, Women's Royal Naval Service during which period she became concerned for the plight of patients with VD and, in particular, the patient who was a single woman and pregnant. No 'respectable' home for unmarried mothers wanted them and treatment then was protracted and tedious. Dorothy Hare set up two hostels for treatment and after-care which continued to be busy until antibiotics made them redundant.

Awarded CBE in 1919. In the same year she became medical registrar at the Royal Free Hospital. She was appointed to the staff of Royal Free and Elizabeth Garrett Anderson Hospitals in 1929.

She sang and drew well; took a keen interest in amateur theatricals; liked to travel. A calm, confident presence.

Oils on canvas, laid down on board, 38¾ by 28⅞ inches, by Frederick John Hayes Whicker, c. 1955

Nearly whole length seated to right, hands in lap, in an interior; light greyish-brown hair, grey eyebrows, pale blue eyes, short prominent nose, short lips, brownish, wrinkled complexion; doctoral hat and scarlet robe lined with purple, over plain black high-necked dress; stool upholstered in brown; light brown wall with dark brown dado below; through the window left is seen the Senate House of London University; signed bottom left: *F. Whicker*.

Presented by Mrs. H. A. T. Child and Mr. Ewan Hare, niece and nephew of the sitter, October 1968.

F. Whicker is the signature of Frederick John Hayes Whicker, of Falmouth, (1956).

126   *Ref: Who's Who in Art*, 8th ed. 1956, pp. 757–758; *Commentary*, April 1969, p. 48.

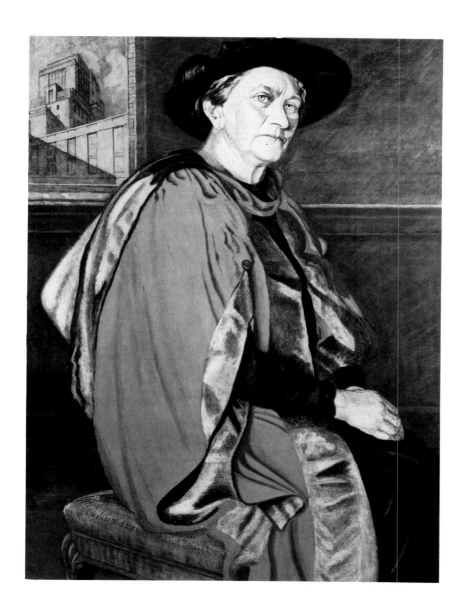

127

Sir Eliab Harvey, MP 1635–1698/9

Born St Laurence Pountney 1635, and educated at Merchant Taylors School. Knighted in 1660, JP and Deputy-Lieutenant for the county of Essex. Was MP for the county from 1678–9; then, for Old Sarum, Wilts. 1679–81, and for Maldon, Essex 1693–8.

Lady Dorothy Harvey 1638–1725/6

(date of birth on portrait almost certainly wrong)

Third daughter of Sir Thomas Whitmore (1st) Bt. – of Shropshire (not to be confused with Sir Thomas Whitmore KB, husband of Anne Whitmore).
Married Sir Eliab Harvey at St Giles-in-the-Fields 1658.

Sir Eliab Harvey

Oils on canvas, 49¾ by 39½ inches, by an unknown artist, 1675

Three-quarter length standing to left, holding brown drapery to chest, his gloved left hand by his side; brown eyebrows, brown eyes, long nose curving downwards, thick lips parted, double chin; mid brown wig parted in centre, touching shoulders, white shirt with broad lace cravat and cuffs, grey velvet coat; crimson silk curtains parted top left, base of column on left on which are the remains of an inscription now very rubbed: *Eliab Harvey | | ,* presumably incorporated in the more recent inscription, bottom left: *Sir Eliab Harvey Kn^t. | Aetatis40. | AD 1675.* Lit from the right.

Property of the Harveian Society of London; on loan to the College, November 1968. From the collection of Sir Francis Whitmore, Orsett Hall, Romford; anonymous property, Christies, 11 December 1964, lot 54, with the portrait of Lady Harvey (see next entry).

This and the companion portrait of Lady Harvey have been incorrectly ascribed to Kneller. They are by a less able hand or hands capable of attractive landscape painting, but weak in figure drawing, and stemming rather from the Lely workshop. It does not seem possible to get closer. A portrait of this Eliab Harvey, or of Eliab, William Harvey's brother, was in the Harvey family collection at Rolls Park, where recorded by Neale. He also appears in the family group of William and Mary Harvey and their three sons.

128   *Ref:* J. P. Neale, *Views of the seats of Noblemen and Gentlemen*, 2nd series, III, 1826.

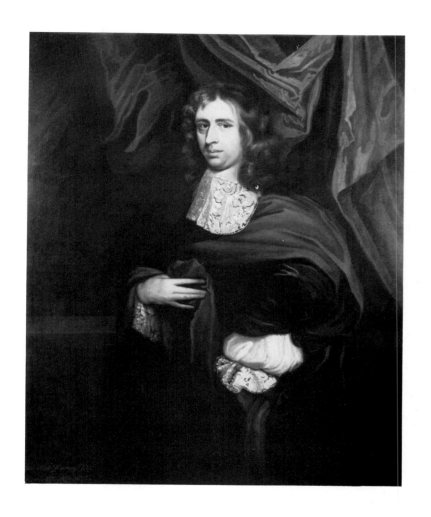

Lady Dorothy Harvey

Oils on canvas, 49 by 29 inches, by an unknown artist, 1675

Nearly whole length seated to right in landscape, and resting her head on her left hand, right hand in lap; curly brown hair, parted in centre, flat on top, a long ringlet falling on either side, deep blue eyes, light brown eyebrows, downward curving nose, full lower lip, slightly pink complexion; single string of pearls at throat, low-cut orange dress, fastened in front with five buckles(?) each of two pearls and a black diamond, similar decoration round her right shoulder, purple drapery; background of rocks and foliage; a distant landscape on right under cloudy pink sky. Inscribed bottom left, in yellow: *Dorothy Harvey | suae (?) AEtatis 33 | Ao. 1675* and in a more recent hand on right: *Daughter of | Sir Thomas Whitmore Bt|Born 1648.*

Property of the Harveian Society of London; loan to the College, November 1968. Like the companion portrait of her husband from the collection of Sir Francis Whitmore, of Orsett Hall, Romford, whose ancestor Sir William Whitmore, 2nd bart. (1627–1699) married the sitter's daughter Mary; Christies, 11 December 1964, lot 54, with the portrait of Sir Eliab Harvey, anonymous property.

130   *Ref:* Burke, *Landed Gentry*, 1952, pp. 2705–06.

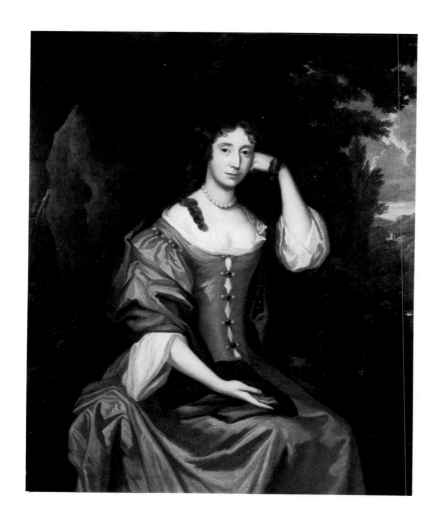

(?) William Harvey 1578–1657 F. 1607

The discoverer of the circulation, outstanding physiologist and inspirer of medical science. Physician to James I and Charles I, he lost the Wardenship of Merton College, Oxford, and his house in London in the Civil War.

(Catalogue I, pp. 202–215)

7. Oils on canvas, 30 by 25 inches, from the studio of Sir Peter Lely

Head and shoulders to left, eyes directed at spectator, hands not shewn; hair beneath tight-fitting black cap, brown eyes, grey eyebrows, tuft moustache and chin, large straight nose, a small pimple by the left nostril; plain white broad hands, black gown; plain brown background, sculpted oval; lit from the right.

Presented in memory of Sir Daniel Davies by his widow, Lady Davies, January 1967.

A typical Lely studio product of the mid 1670s; perhaps, on comparison with authentic portraits, intended for a posthumous representation of Harvey, but the liveliness suggests rather another unidentified sitter painted from life. From the dress, the sitter might equally be a divine or lawyer.

Ref: Catalogue I, 1964, pp. 202–15; *Annals*, 26 January 1967, p. 6f.

132   *(See also Medals pp. 208–211)*

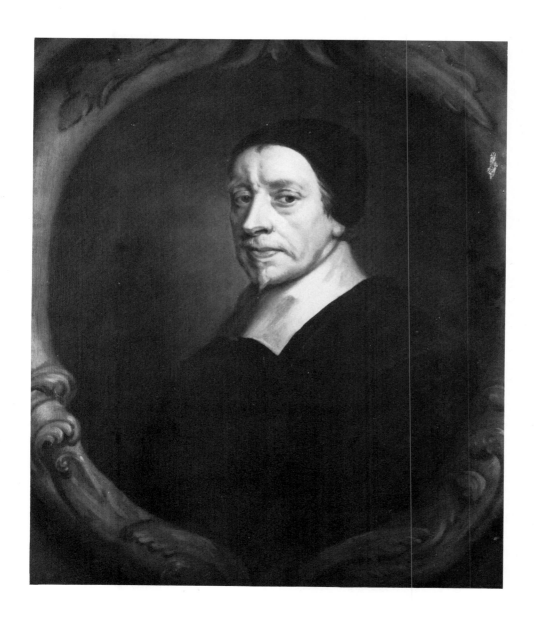

William Hunter 1718–1783 L. 1756

Scottish born anatomist, surgeon and midwife, who became one of the great teachers and practitioners in London, forming a superb library and collections of medals and natural history specimens. Elder brother of John Hunter.

(Catalogue I, pp. 230–235)

4. Enamel miniature, 1⅜ by 1¼ inches, by an unknown artist

Head and shoulders to left, head turned towards spectator; brown eyebrows, blue eyes; bushy grey wig touching shoulders, black solitaire, white neckband and shirt ruffle, bright blue coat with long gold button-holes; green background.

Presented by Miss Angela Oliver, 1972.

John Bogle exhibited a miniature of 'the late Dr. W. Hunter' at the R.A. in 1785, as did W. Brown. Neither is known to have worked in enamel; William Brown was a gem engraver. Our miniature seems to be taken from Ramsay's portrait of Hunter, but is closer to the copy presented to the College in 1829 than to the original painted *c.* 1760, in the Hunterian collection, Glasgow University.

Ref: R.A. catalogue 1785 (281, 362); *Catalogue* I, 1964, pp. 230 ff.; *Annals*, 27 April 1972, p. 90a.

134

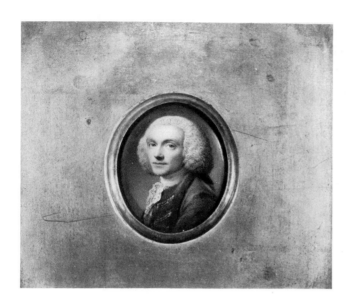

5. Oils on canvas, 30 ½ by 25 ¼ inches, ? by James Barry, c. 1784

Half length seated, eyes directed to right, his right hand in coat, left hand on arm of chair; white wig, brown eyebrows, dark brown eyes, sunken cheeks, pursed lower lip; white neckband and shirt front, and wrist ruffles, dark blue(?) coat, green upholstered chair; plain brown background, lit from the right. On back on bottom bar of relining stretcher an early manuscript label: *William Hunter M.D. F.R.S. | Believed to be by Pine.*

Presented by Miss Angela Oliver, 1972.

The type is not by Pine but by James Barry, and relates to the head of Hunter in the series of murals illustrating the *Progress of Human Culture* painted for the Great Room of the Society of Arts in the Adelphi 1777–1783. Hunter is introduced into the Fifth Picture: *The Distribution of Premiums in the Society of Arts* and is next to the Duke of Northumberland, the Earl of Radnor and William Locke. Though clearly early, it is hard to judge in its present condition whether our portrait precedes or follows the group: the only comparable known work, the study for the head of Samuel Johnson, N.P.G. 1185, is much more incisive, but this has recently been cleaned.

Ref: J. Barry, *Works*, II, 1809, pp. 340–41; E. K. Waterhouse, *Painting in Britain 1530–1790* (Pelican History of British Art), 1969, p. 189.

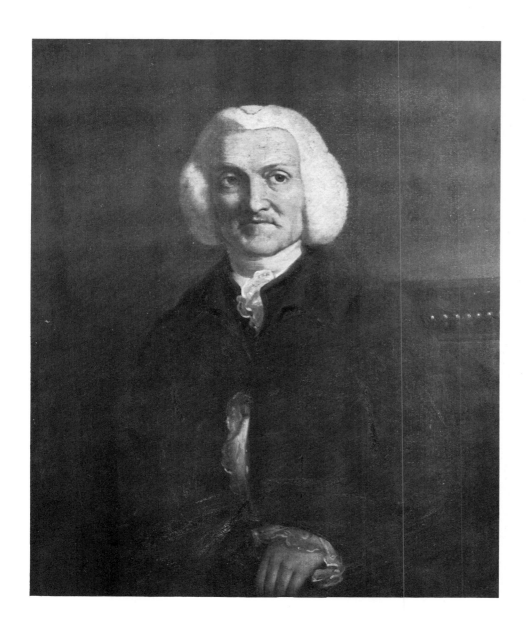

137

Geoffrey Hales Jennings 1905– F. 1949

Retired now and living in Sussex.

Born in Horsham, Sussex, the son of a schoolmaster. Educated at Christ's Hospital; Cambridge; St Mary's Hospital. Senior physician to the Edgware General Hospital, 1951–63 Member, Board of Governors, National Heart Hospital. Wrote '*Arteritis of the Temporal Vessels*' – the first paper to be published in Europe on the subject – and numerous other papers.

Athletic in his youth – a keen cricketer and rugby player; artistic – one of his great loves is opera; he has written several opera libretti, and he has had poetry published in *The Field* magazine; he also likes photography and painting in water colours.

Oils on canvas, 30 by 25 inches, by Patrick Edward Phillips, 1958

Half length seated to left, hands clasped in lap; short, greying hair, grey eyebrows, pale blue eyes, horn rim spectacles, long lips, firm chin; white striped collar, plain blue tie, scarlet M.D. gown over blue jacket; wooden chair, plain blue background, lighter to left; lit from right. Signed bottom right *Phillips*. On the back, the label of the Royal Society of Portrait Painters where it was exhibited 1958.

Presented by the sitter, 1970, who commissioned it as a record of the first consultant physician at Edgware General Hospital.

Pentimenti down the right side of his face, indicating that it has been turned more towards the spectator.

Ref: Catalogue of R.S.P.P. 1958 (4); als, from the donor, 4, 21 June 1970; *Annals*, 28 January 1971, p. 12b.

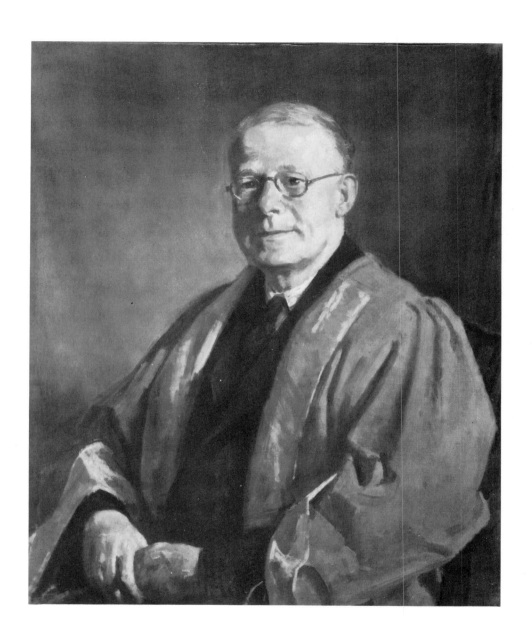

139

John Latham 1761–1843 F. 1789 P. 1813–1819

A hard-working, conscientious and religious man, of uncertain health, who did great service to the College, particularly in regard to its library.

(Catalogue I, pp. 254–255)

2. Miniature, watercolours on ivory, 3 ¼ by 2⁹⁄₁₆ inches, oval by Alexander Pope

Head and shoulders, seated slightly to right; straight grey hair, covering ears, grey eyebrows, light grey eyes, large nose, long upper lip, firm jaw, pale complexion; white cravat tied in large bow, brownish purple double-breasted coat, white waistcoat with yellow stripe; chair upholstered in scarlet cloth, grey background. An early manuscript label on the back of the contemporary frame: *John Latham MD, FRS. | born 1761, died 1843. | Painted about 1806, | by Alexander Pope, Comedian. | G (?). Q (?).*

Bequeathed by Miss R. E. Ormerod, December 1959, and lent to Mrs. J. C. Wilford, March 1960.

Alexander Pope 1763–1835, born in Cork, was a pupil of the pastel painter H. D. Hamilton. He painted mainly miniatures, and acted in Dublin and London. His first two wives, both actresses, died young. His third was the widow of the painter Francis Wheatley. He had some celebrated sitters, including Mrs. Siddons.

Ref: Annals, 28 January 1960, p. 114d; al. to Mrs. J. C. Wilford 11 March 1960; *Catalogue* I, 1964, pp. 244–45; D. Foskett, *A Dictionary of British Miniaturists,* I, 1972, pp. 453–54.

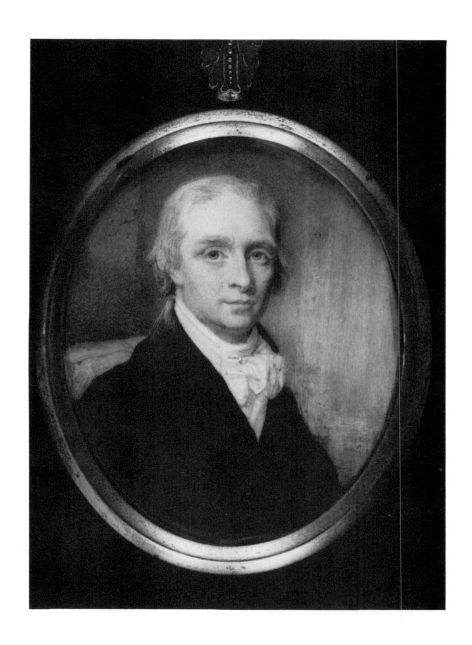

141

John Coakley Lettsom 1744–1815 L. 1770

One of a pair of twins, the only children to survive of seven sets of twins born to his mother, Lettsom was born on the island of Little Vandyke, nr. Tortola, in the Virgin Islands. En route to school in England he was befriended by a preacher who was the brother of Dr John Fothergill, and who later became his guardian.

Lettsom served his apprenticeship in Yorkshire, afterwards returning to the estate on Little Vandyke that had passed to him on his brother's death, and his first act was to free all the slaves – an act which left him penniless. However, he managed to save enough money from his practice on Tortola to return again to England.

He attended the lectures of Dr Cullen in Edinburgh on fever – a subject of particular interest to him – and in his first publication drew on a number of Dr Cullen's ideas and opinions without, unfortunately, revealing his source. Through the patronage of Dr Fothergill and Lettsom's co-religionists from the Society of Friends, he built up a very substantial practice in London – the largest, indeed, in the city. And he also had the good fortune to marry a woman of means. But although rich, he was a philanthropist and spent money lavishly, and consequently was never in a position to retire.

A rather curious interest of his was the mangel-wurzel which he was very keen to have introduced into this country. He did his best to promote the vegetable – grew it himself, imported it and distributed it, and translated a French pamphlet about it called 'An Account of the Mangel-Wurzel, or Root of Scarcity'. Other interests included the eradication of intemperance; beekeeping; prison reform; and he wrote voluminously, much of it apparently done in his carriage en route to and from his patients. Not known to be an outstanding physician, it is mainly as a philanthropist and as peacemaker in the quarrels of his medical colleagues that he is remembered. With the intention of bringing together in companionship physicians, apothecaries and surgeons, Lettsom was the principal founder, in 1773, of the Medical Society of London.

Medallion, pink wax, 4 ¼ inches diameter by T. R. Poole, 1809

Bust in profile to left; large straight nose, double chin; wig with two rows of curls over ear, shirt ruffle, two buttons of coat seen below; incised *Dr. Lettsom* / and signed and dated Poole 1809 on the cutaway; dark brown glass background. On the back of the contemporary frame, Poole's trade label, on which has been written *John Coakley Lettsom MD LD DCL ... President of the Medical Society.*

Source and date of acquisition unknown.

Our wax is evidently the source of the engraving 'from a model' by W. Skelton published in 1817 as the frontispiece to Pettigrew's *Memoirs* of Lettsom. Another version belongs to his great-great grandson, J. H. A. Elliott. Lettsom addresses a group of the 'Institutors of the

Medical Society of London' painted by S. Medley, and engraved by R. Wilkinson, 1801; a separate portrait by Medley was engraved by W. Ridley, *c.* 1803; both portraits are still in the possession of the Society. Another small engraving by T. Holloway was published in the *European Magazine* 1787. A group ascribed to Zoffany, showing Lettsom and his family in the grounds of Grove Hill, *c.* 1775, is now in the Wellcome Institute.

Ref: Dictionary of National Biography, XI, 1909, p. 1015; O'Donoghue, III, 1912, pp. 53–54, V, 1922, pp. 60–61; J. J. Abraham, *Lettsom: His Life, Time, Friends and Descendants*, 1933, p. 438; T. Hunt, *The Medical Society of London*, 1972, frontispiece and title-page and pp. 22–35; Burgess, 1973, p. 214 and references there given; E. J. Pyke, *A Biographical Dictionary of Wax Modellers*, 1973, pp. 112–13.

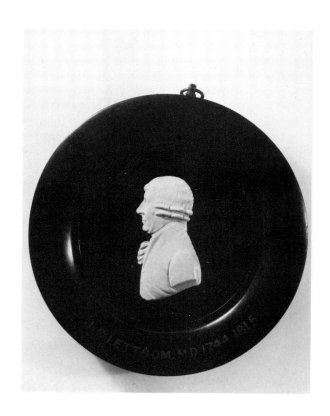

Jean Andre De Luc 1727–1817

Born in Geneva; educated by his father, who distrusted rationalism and taught his son to do so.

Jean De Luc became a merchant and politician, but when his business failed he moved to England. Geology had long been a serious 'hobby' with him and his appointment as reader to George III's wife, Queen Charlotte, provided him both with security and the freedom to pursue his researches.

He attempted to explain phenomena in terms of the Old Testament. As well as geology, he was interested in meteorology and in 1771 published the first correct rules for measuring the heights of mountains barometrically. He invented the 'dry pile' – a method of producing an electric current.

Because he had always to be near the Queen, he lived at Windsor and, after being confined to his home by illness for a number of years, he died there.

Oils on panel, 11 ½ by 9 ½ inches, by an unknown artist, c. 1816

Half length facing spectator, holding steel folding spectacles in his right hand; curly grey hair, full at sides, bald on top, pale brown eyes, light arched eyebrows, large nose, thin lips; black coat with turned down collar, black waistcoat, white shirt; plain brown background. Inscribed on the back of the panel: *J A De Luc. F.R.S. | Died November 1817* (sic) *aged 91. | This portrait was painted | about a year before his death.*

A drawing by C. Penny is known by his engraving; a portrait by W. de Stetten was engraved by Schroeder, and a painting by H. Wyatt was engraved by P. Audinet.

144   *Ref:* O'Donoghue, II, 1910, p. 30; Burgess, 1973, p. 96.

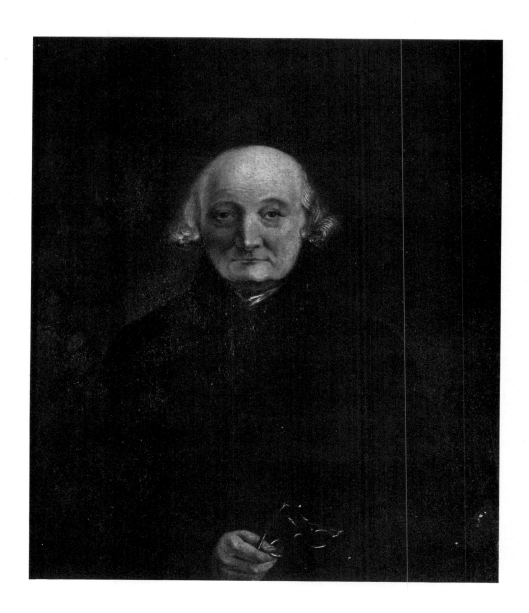

William MacMichael 1784–1839 F. 1818

A banker's son, William MacMichael was born in Shropshire and educated at Bridgnorth Grammar School; Christchurch, Oxford; Edinburgh under Alexander Munro; and St Bartholomew's where Abernethy was active. In 1811 he was awarded a Radcliffe travelling fellowship and this enabled him to see such romantic and mysterious places as Greece, Turkey, Bulgaria, Rumania, Russia, Sweden, and Austria, where he acted as physician to the British Ambassador. He graduated DM from Oxford in 1816 and then had two further years of travel, described in his *Journey from Moscow to Constantinople*, with illustrations by himself.

Twice he was Censor for the College, in 1820 and again in 1832, and he held the office of Registrar for five years from 1824, and was Consilarius in 1836. While physician to the Middlesex Hospital, he was, thanks to his friend and patron, Sir Henry Halford, appointed physician-extraordinary to George IV in 1829. The following year saw him as William IV's librarian, and the next, as physician-in-ordinary to the king. King William gave him his own gold-headed cane, saying that since MacMichael had cured him of gout he no longer needed it. In 1827 MacMichael cleverly and delightfully used the device of ownership of Radcliffe's cane to write brief biographies of Radcliffe, Mead, Askew, William and David Pitcairn and Baillie, in *The Gold-Headed Cane* (reproduced in facsimile in 1968 by the RCP).

William MacMichael was fond of society and society was fond of him. His easy-going disposition and fund of anecdotes from his adventures abroad made him an attractive personality.

In 1837 he was struck down by a stroke and compelled to retire, so that he did not attend King William at his death in that year, and two years later he died.

Watercolours on white paper, 11$\frac{15}{16}$ by 9$\frac{3}{4}$ inches, by William Haines, 1823

Short half length seated to right, head and eyes turned towards spectator; receding curly grey hair cut short, large brown eyebrows, greyish blue eyes, dimpled chin, fresh complexion; white collar and stock, double (?) breasted grey coat, matching waistcoat; armchair lightly outlined in pencil, stippled light grey background to right of body, lit from left. Faintly signed and dated in pencil, bottom right: *W. Haines P^t / Aug 1823*. Modern labels on the back giving biographical details of the sitter and the name of a former owner J. Cheese (?) N(?)ewby.

The gift of Miss Joan Cheese, great-grand-daughter of the sitter, and Mrs. Mary Hindle.

Ref: Annals, 25 July 1974, Doc. 17a.

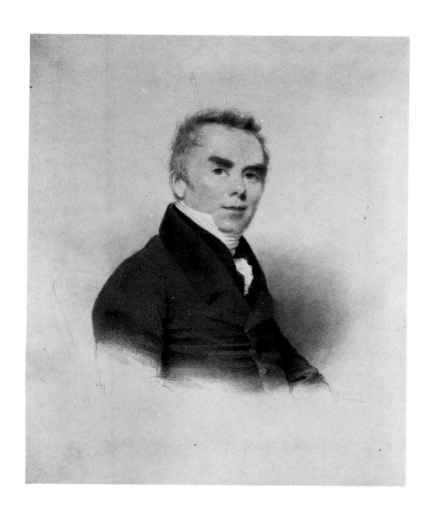

Sir Arthur MacNalty 1880–1969 F. 1930

This quiet, scholarly man will be remembered both for his work in public health and preventive medicine, and for his numerous historical publications, which included *Henry VIII: a Difficult Patient*.

In 1908, with Sir Thomas Lewis, he recorded for the first time the use of the electrocardiograph in diagnosing heart disease. For 5½ years from 1935 he was Chief Medical Officer to the Ministry of Health and Board of Education, having joined the Ministry originally in 1919. In 1940, thanks to MacNalty, anti-diphtheria vaccine was made available free to local authorities. His recommendations, contained in his report on infant measles and pneumonia, were adopted by the Local Government Board and, in consequence, there was a noticeable reduction in the mortality rate. From 1937–40 he was hon. physician to George VI. He helped to organize the emergency medical services for World War II and from 1941, at the invitation of Churchill, was Editor-in-Chief of the official *Medical History of the War*, a monumental work that he lived to see completed.

Other instances of the fascination that medical history had for him were his Hon. Presidency of the British Society for History of Medicine and his role as an official historian of the RCP's College Club. The Tudor period was the one in which he specialized, but his writings were by no means confined to one period and, indeed, among other things, he wrote a biography of Walter Scott, translated the odes of Horace and was the author of *A Book of Crimes*.

A friend of Monckton Copeman, he gave the first Monckton Copeman Lecture when an old man in his 80s.

Always quiet and self-effacing and, it is suggested, underestimated, he was nonetheless a very determined man. First and foremost. MacNalty was a scholar who liked such quiet pursuits as fishing, boating, philately and painting, but medical history was clearly his great and abiding love.

Oils on canvas, 30 by 24 inches, by Clare Collas, 1958

Half length, looking to right, his left hand on jacket, body fronting spectator; smooth grey hair, light grey-brown, pale blue eyes, long thin lips, rather pale complexion; white collar and shirt, black tie, black gown with scarlet hood over single-breasted black coat and waistcoat; bookshelves behind; lit from the right. Signed, bottom right in red, *C. Collas*.

Bequeathed by the sitter, October 1969.

148 *Ref:* Annals, 30 October 1969, p. 164b.

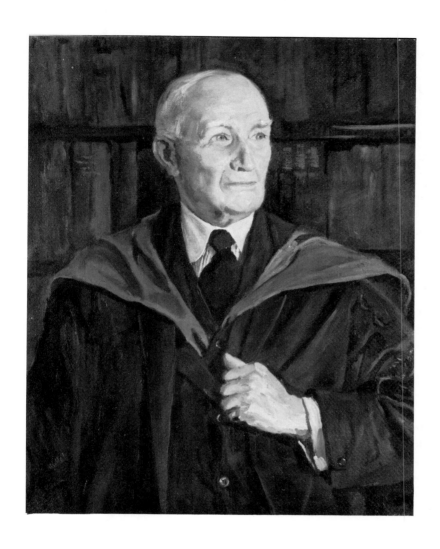

149

William Murray, 1st Earl of Mansfield 1705–1793

Born at the Abbey of Scone, William Murray was fourth son of the 5th Viscount Stormont, and was educated at Perth Grammar school, Westminster (where he was King's scholar), and Christ Church, Oxford. Younger son of an impoverished Scottish peer, he was destined for the Church, but was assisted by a friend Thomas Foley (later Baron Foley) to read law.

An early talent for declamation was studiously rehearsed, sometimes in front of his friend Alexander Pope. Lifelong enmity with Pitt (Earl of Chatham) began when Murray beat Pitt for a Latin poem prize at Oxford.

Called to the Bar at Lincoln's Inn in 1730, KC and solicitor-general 1742, attorney-general 1754 and Lord Chief Justice 1756 – turning down the Duchy of Lancaster and a pension of £6000 offered to him to stay in the Commons, where he was an outstanding leader.

Macaulay described him as 'the father of modern toryism'. In American affairs he was wholly for coercion and when he failed to inspire a coalition to cope with the situation, he retired from politics.

Famous cases included his refusal to allow prosecutions against Roman Catholic priests for saying mass, which carried the penalty of life imprisonment. Mansfield freed the West Indian slave, James Somersett, in 1771 on grounds that slavery was 'so odious' that nothing could 'be suffered to support it'. He was the first to allow a Quaker to affirm in place of taking an oath. A sincere Christian, he would nevertheless have tried a case on Good Friday if counsel had not pointed out that he would be following a precedent set by Pontius Pilate. Although a victim of the Gordon riots – his house was wrecked – he tried Lord George Gordon with strict impartiality.

In the struggles between the RCP and its licentiates, 1767–1771. Mansfield accepted the distinction between fellows and licentiates, but warned the College to review its statutes and not to make admission so narrow that even a Boerhaave resident in London would be excluded.

At his·request he was buried in the North Cross, Westminster Abbey, near the scene of his early education.

William Murray, 1st Earl of Mansfield (formerly called John Arbuthnot by Charles Jervas, c. 1715) by J. Vanloo, c. 1738

Despite its inscription, as Gibson points out our portrait proves to represent Mansfield. It is too young a man, too late to represent Arbuthnot, and is a version of the earlier portrait by Vanloo, with the same face but in a wig, engraved by Basire as painted in 1732. A fine Kit-cat size version still in Lord Clarendon's collection belonged to his ancestor, the sitter's friend, Henry Cornbury and Baron Hyde, 1710–1753, who was also painted by Vanloo. It is listed in his catalogue of 1750: *Lord Hyde's Dressing Room ... MR. SOLICITOR-GENERAL MURRAY.*

Ref: Catalogue I, 1964, pp. 28–29; R. Gibson, *Catalogue of Pictures in the Collection of the Earl of Clarendon*, 1977, (51), (96), and refs. there cited.

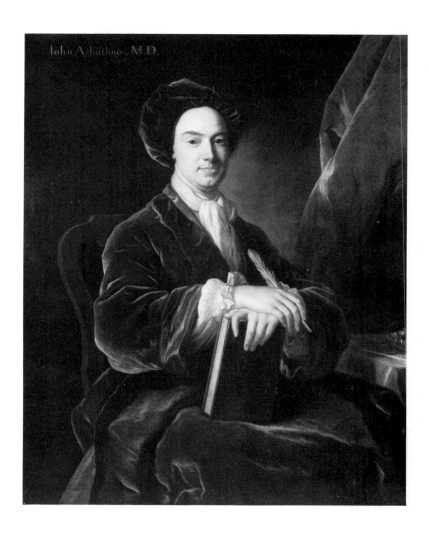

Sir Theodore de Mayerne 1573–1655 F. 1616

A Protestant born in Geneva, de Mayerne was one of the first to use chemical remedies including mercury. He refused to conform to the Catholic Church in France and came to England where he achieved great distinction, became physician to the Royal family, and was elected Fellow of the College at a special Comitia called for the purpose.

(Catalogue I, pp. 276–279)

3. Oils on canvas, 13¼ by 11¼ inches, by an unknown artist after Sir Peter Paul Rubens

Nearly whole length seated, head tilted to his right, hands in lap; white hair, dark eyes, long drooping moustache and beard; white collar and cuffs, black robes, dark green sleeve, scarlet chair; landscape seen through window, plain black background.

Presented by Mrs. Douglas Hearn, October 1966.

Our oil is a simplified reduction from the portrait taken by Rubens about 1630, discussed in the previous volume. It follows the North Carolina oil, but omitting the statue of Aesculapius. It seems to be eighteenth century work, and could derive either from an engraving or from an oil of the North Carolina type. One, conceivably N.P.G. 1652, was in Dr. Mead's collection.

Ref: D. T. Piper, *Catalogue of the Seventeenth-Century Portraits in the National Portrait Gallery,* 1963, p. 229; *Catalogue I,* 1964, pp. 276–79; *Annals,* 27 October 1966, p. 247.

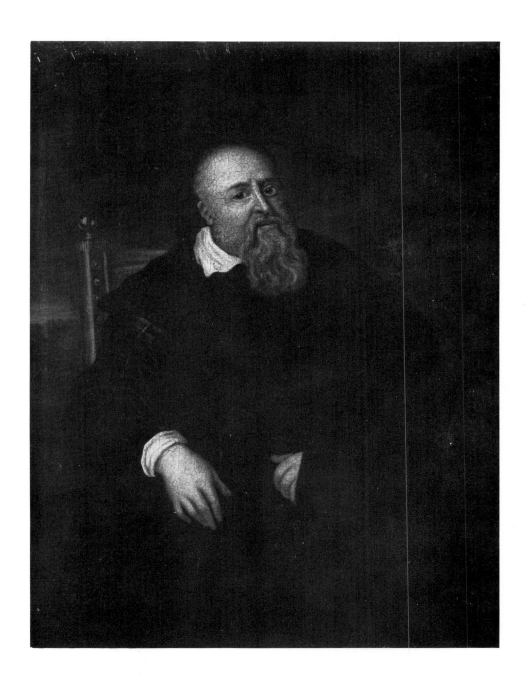

153

Charles Mitchell 1783–1856

Naval surgeon. While he was surgeon on board the flagship Vigo, based at St. Helena, Charles Mitchell was called in to consult with Shortt, Arnott and Antommarchi about the condition – then grave – of Napoleon, but he never actually saw the patient alive. He was, however, present at the post-mortem examination of Napoleon and signed the official report.

Retired to the Isle of Wight and died there aged 73.

Oils on canvas, 37¼ by 28⅛ inches, by an unknown artist

Half length to right, lorgnette in his right hand, his left hand resting on base of column; close-cut dark brown hair parted on right, brown side whiskers, lighter brown eyebrows, pale blue eyes, full lower lip, chin clean-shaven, fresh complexion; white collar and shirt, broad black neckband, black coat, open, black waistcoat; dark brown background, lighter to right. On the back of the canvas, a stamp: *Prepared | by | J.H.SIMPSON | ARTIST COLOUR-MAN | 54 | LONDON ROAD | Southw[ark?]*

On indefinite loan from J. C. Medley.

The hand has not been identified, but is not far from Stephen Pearce, who had a number of medical and naval sitters.

154   *Ref:* Annals, 30 April 1964, p. 179.

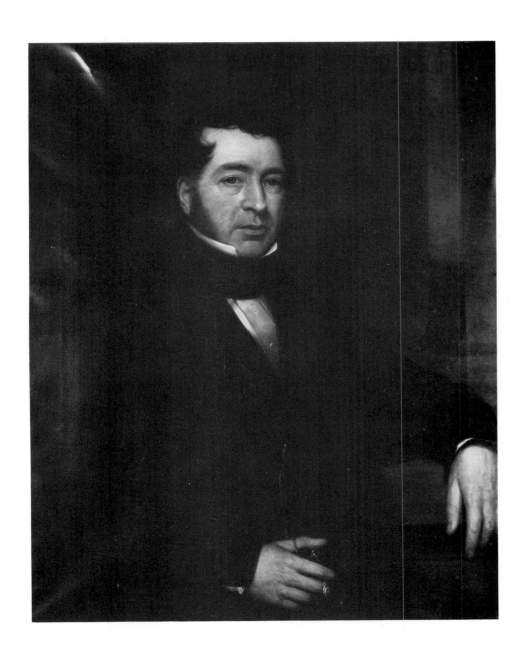

Charles McMoran Wilson, 1st Baron Moran of Manton 1883– F. 1921 P. 1941–50

Born in Skipton, Yorkshire, the son of Dr John Forsythe Wilson. Knighted 1938; made a baron 1943. Physician to Winston Churchill for 25 years, from 1940–65. Churchill said of him that he was 'the man who saved my life'.

Obtained the Military Cross through his work in the Battle of the Somme during World War I. Entry from the *BMJ* (*II*, 1916 Sept. 30 p. 471): 'Temporary Captain C. McM. Wilson MD RAMC – For conspicuous gallantry and devotion to duty during operations. He worked for over an hour digging out wounded men, at great personal risk. He then returned to his aid post and attended to the wounded. Later, hearing that an officer had been wounded, he passed through 100 yards of the enemy's artillery barrage, dressed his wounds, and finally got him into safety as soon as the barrage permitted. On other occasions he has done fine and gallant work'.

In 1945 the popular and highly successful *Anatomy of Courage* was published. It is a non-technical psychological analysis of courage in a modern army, based upon Lord Moran's experiences in the two world wars. He believed that courage was self-willed, a conscious act of decision, not an accidental gift of nature, and that it could wear out: that to preserve it, rest was vital.

He has always been very concerned about medical education. From his Address as President of the RCP in 1941, he said: 'We have to extirpate this blind cult of memory and the stored fact. We have to ask how the quick curiosity of the average child has been converted into the dull drudge we so often encounter in the finals ...'

He was Dean of St Mary's Hospital Medical School from 1920–1945, a guiding spirit throughout a period of development and change.

Lord Moran was against the National Health Service because he thought it would interfere with the freedom of doctors, and he was worried also that the Government might be trying to get medical service 'on the cheap'. He was Chairman (the first) of the Distinction Awards Committee, 1949.

He answered questions anonymously on the BBC's Brains Trust: intellectual, 'pale, ascetic'; religious – and, being something of a puritan, he probably disapproved of Churchill's self-indulgence; loves the country, hates cities.

The highly controversial diaries (*Winston Churchill, The Struggle for Survival*, published in 1966) made him an almost notorious figure. Ironically, in 1950, a piece from *The Sunday Times* (January 15) Portrait Gallery read as follows: 'No statesman's observations on the great men and events with which he was brought into contact would be more valuable than Lord Moran's, or wiser.' Moran's diaries caused a furore, which he must have foreseen. He himself justified them by saying that 'it is not possible to follow the last 25 years of Sir Winston's life without a knowledge of his medical background. It was exhaustion of mind and body that accounted for much that is otherwise inexplicable in the last year of the war, for instance the deterioration in his relations with President Roosevelt. ... and in justice to him ought not to be left out of his story. ... I may add that I told Sir Winston about what I proposed to do'. (Letter to *The Times* 25/4/66.) (The diaries were published 15 months after Churchill's death.) In a later letter, 2/6/66, Lord Moran said Winston Churchill approved, saying he was sure he would like whatever he wrote about him.

One is bound to wonder what Lord Moran's motives were in publishing the diaries so soon after Churchill's death. Perhaps Moran's publish-and-be-damned attitude showed in him a certain courage (a motive in itself, even?).

Lord Moran]

Oils on board, 24 by 19½ inches, by Pietro Annigoni, 1951

Head and shoulders, head tilted to left, but looking up to right, body to left, the thumb of his left hand marking place in an open book; receding grey hair, wrinkled forehead, thin light brown eyebrows, blue eyes, pale complexion; President's gown of gold lace on black, white collar, black tie, black coat and waistcoat; window-like blue background, brown panelling; book bound in scarlet morocco. Signed on the panelling level with his right shoulder: *P. ANNIGONI* / monogram / *.LI.* / *LONDRA*.

Commissioned for the College, 1951, and received 1974. A replica was presented to the sitter by the College. The original was exhibited at the Royal Academy.

Presumably the portrait exhibited at the Royal Academy 1952; exhibited Wildenstein 1954 (23), their label on the back, and lent by the sitter to the Annigoni exhibition 1961 (8). Juliet Pannett exhibited a portrait at the Royal Society of Portrait Painters 1960.

Ref: R. A. catalogue 1952 (802); R.S.P.P. catalogue 1960 (231); *BMJ*, 21 July 1951; *Who's Who in Art*, 16th ed., 1972, p. 617.

158

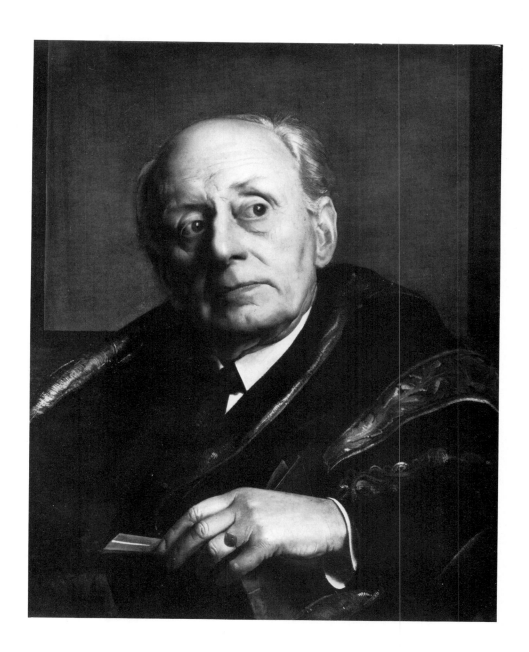

159

Charles Murchison 1830–79 F. 1859

Born in Jamaica, the son of the Hon. Alexander Murchison MD; raised in Scotland; educated at Aberdeen University, where he was an arts student, then Edinburgh, where he read medicine with distinction.

His first post was as physician to the British Embassy in Turin. From 1853–55 he was Professor of Chemistry at Calcutta Medical College and during this period he accompanied an expedition to Burma. Soon after his return to England he was appointed physician first at King's College Hospital, then the Middlesex, with a second appointment at the London Fever Hospital, where he edited the reports for many years. Finally he came to the fore as a brilliant clinical teacher at St Thomas's.

Before he died, he was physician-in-ordinary to the Duke and Duchess of Connaught. Suffered from a serious heart disease for years but was determined to continue working. He died, in fact, in his consulting room, having just seen the last of the day's patients.

Charles Murchison was a man with very solid – what are thought of as 'typically British' qualities; honest, thorough, with plain manners; a reliable friend – a man one felt one could trust. He liked geology, natural history, fishing.

The Murchison scholarship in medicine was established in his memory and is administered each year alternately by the RCP and Edinburgh University.

Chalk and wash on paper, in an oval mount, 25⅞ by 20 inches, by Henry Joseph Fradelle

Head and shoulders to left; blackish-brown hair brushed close, side whiskers, brown eyes, and eyebrows, drooping moustache on upper lip, curly beard, pale complexion; white shirt with narrow slate-coloured cravat, grey coat open over double-breasted waistcoat with wide lapels. Signed *Fradelle* above his right forearm.

Presented by the sitter's grandson, Dr. A. M. Humphry, October 1964.

Fradelle died in London in 1865, but the portrait may antedate this by a few years; the only other likeness available for comparison is the marble bust, for St. Thomas's Hospital, by E. Roscoe Mullins, exhibited Royal Academy 1881, and which may have been posthumous. Stephen Pearce exhibited a portrait at the Royal Academy in 1871. A lithograph after Fradelle lettered 'Portrait de Murchison' is dated 1849 but represents Sir Roderick Impey Murchison, 1792–1871, on comparison with authentic portraits.

Ref: R.A. catalogues 1871 (1109), 1881 (1471); U. Thieme and F. Becker, *Allgemeine Lexikon der bildenden Kunstler*, XII, 1916, p. 272; al. from donor, 16 May 1964; *Annals*, 30 July 1964, p. 229.

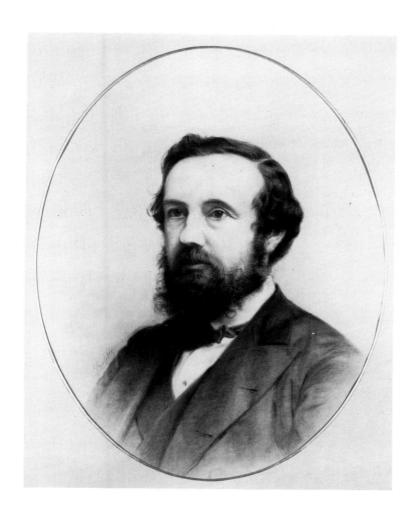

William Murray 1839–1920 F. 1872

William Murray's career was mainly spent in his native North. He died in Cumberland, having married twice and fathered three sons – one of whom was G. R. Murray FRCP – and five daughters.

His early education was at Durham School but his medical education seems to have been of a rather peripatetic nature – Edinburgh, Newcastle, University College London, and Paris. In 1859 he qualified, and his first house appointment was at University College Hospital. From 1864–78 he lectured on physiology at Newcastle School of Medicine. He helped to found the Hospital for Sick Children there, and held appointments at several local hospitals. Although first and foremost Murray was a paediatrician and a gynaecologist, he was one of the first to treat abdominal aneurysm successfully by pressure.

Said to have been a man of 'strong personality', he was religious and one of his activities was to deliver lunchtime talks on religion to factory-workers. He also enjoyed such countryside pursuits as shooting and fishing, retiring to live close to his favourite river, the Eden.

The image one is left with is of a thorough-going Victorian, a man very much the product of his time.

Oils on canvas, 30 by 24 inches, by his daughter Dorothy Lever Murray

Almost whole length standing to left and looking down, his left hand in pocket; curly white hair, bald on top, white side whiskers, dark eyes and eyebrows, straight nose, pointed chin, fresh complexion; soft white collar, black tie, grey jacket with red and blue handkerchief, brown pullover with green and brown pattern, matching grey plus fours, dark brown socks, brown background. Signed with initials bottom left *D.L.M.*, and in full, bottom right, *D. L. Murray*.

Presented by Miss D. L. Murray, 1972, her exhibition label on the back.

The artist exhibited the portrait at City of Carlisle Art Gallery, 1962.

162 *Ref:* Correspondence with Miss D. L. Murray 1972; *Annals*, 27 April 1972, p. 90a.

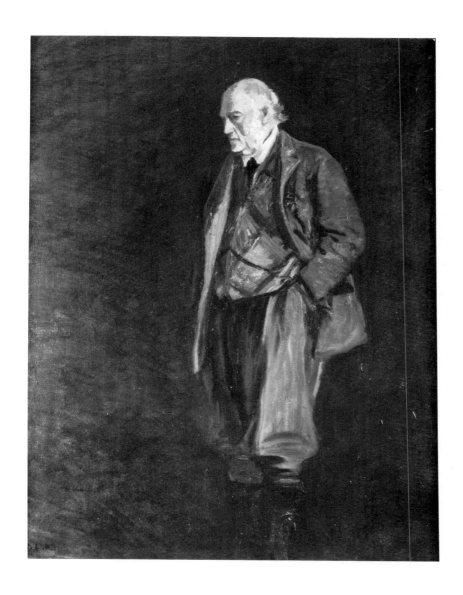

Henry Percy, 9th Earl of Northumberland
1564–1632

Born at Tynemouth Castle, eldest son of the eighth Earl, Henry Percy was early educated in the protestant faith. Later during a visit to Paris he came under suspicion of sharing the views of catholic friends. He succeeded his father in 1585. His main interests were in alchemy and astrology and through his scientific experiments he became known as 'the Wizard Earl'. He was installed as a Knight of the Garter in 1596 and in 1599 bore the insignia of the Garter to Henry IV of France.

The Earl was an irascible, quarrelsome man and a harsh landlord. His marriage to Dorothy, sister of the second Earl of Essex, was uncongenial to both of them. He became strongly addicted to tobacco – he made many protests about the imprisonment of Sir Walter Raleigh – and lost large sums in gambling.

When James VI of Scotland came to the English throne, Northumberland ingratiated himself with the King and, although no avowed catholic, sought and obtained assurances of toleration for English catholics.

On November 4 1605 he received his kinsman Thomas Percy for dinner at Syon House. The next day the Gunpowder Plot was discovered and Thomas Percy incriminated as one of the chief conspirators. Despite Northumberland's protests of disinterest in religion and politics, he was brought before the Star Chamber Court and sentenced to pay £30,000, to lose all offices and be kept in the Tower for life. Eventually he paid £11,000 and stayed in the Tower, where he employed a staff in studies of military fortification, astrology and medicine, for 16 years, emerging with defiant splendour to pass the remaining eleven years of his life at Petworth, where he and his wife are buried.

Oils on canvas, 50 ½ by 40 ½ inches, after Sir Anthony Van Dyck

Nearly whole length, seated, head resting on his right hand; dark brown hair with quiff on top, receding over temples, dark brown eyes, dark brown moustache and full beard; plain white collar and cuffs, black gown with gold frogging; white paper on table left, a curtain behind, column on right.

Given by Dr. C. E. Kellett, 1975.

An old, relined, copy of Van Dyck's original at Petworth (223) where the sitter was buried; there are reproductions at Castle Howard and in Lord Denbigh's collection. Dr. Kellett bought his version from Andersons and Garland in 1935; its previous history is not known, but it is probably seventeenth or early eighteenth century work and possibly from a North country house. The date of the original is not known, but if from life, should be either 1621 or 1632, the only years in which sitter and artist are likely to have met. An earlier whole length, ascribed to Mytens (Petworth 590, repetition or copy at Alnwick) is near the engraving by Francis Delaram, 1619 (Hind 27): its true date is probably *c.* 1602 as it has an inscription alluding to Northumberland's service in the Low Countries. Another engraving by Delaram

(Hind 26) shews the sitter in a hat: it was afterwards altered to represent Ernest Count Mansfield. Miniatures by Isaac Oliver of a Knight of the Garter in the Fitzwilliam Museum and the Rijksmuseum though alike are not necessarily both of the same person, and may represent either Northumberland or the Earl of Mulgrave.

Ref: C. H. Collins Baker, *Catalogue of the Petworth Collection*, 1920, pp. 29, 86, and pls. facing; A. M. Hind, *Engraving in England*, II, 1955, pp. 228–29, and pl. 131; V. & A. *Hilliard and Oliver*, exhibition catalogue, 1947 (152, 168); *Annals*, 29 January 1976, Doc. 6.

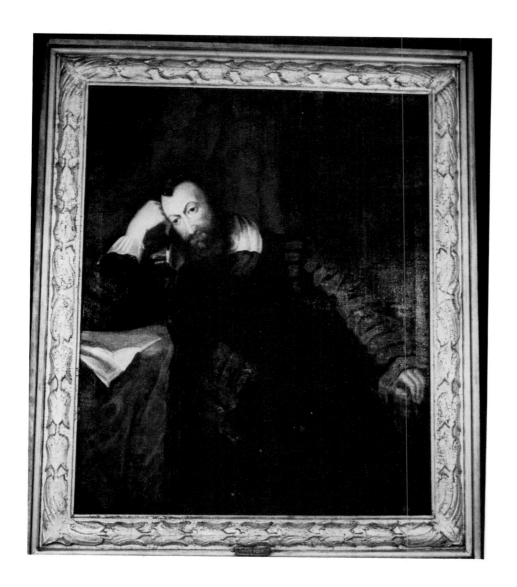

Christopher Robert Pemberton 1765–1822 F. 1796

Grandson of a Lord Chief Justice, Christopher Pemberton was born in Cambridge-shire and educated at Bury St Edmund's and Caius College, Cambridge. He was Censor in 1796, 1804 and 1811, delivered the Goulstonian Lecture in 1797 and the Harveian Oration in 1806. A Fellow of the Royal Society, he was appointed physician-extraordinary to the king, and from 1800–08 physician to St George's Hospital. Sadly it became impossible for him to carry on; he suffered from tic douloureux and no treatment of the day offered any alleviation from the terrible pain, though Sir Astley Cooper tried dividing several branches of the 5th nerve. Pemberton bore it bravely but retired at last to Kent, where death came to his rescue suddenly, in the form of a stroke, at the age of 57.

Sarah Pemberton

First wife of C. R. Pemberton. Maiden name and dates of marriage and death unknown. In August 1794 Pemberton married Eleanor, daughter of James Hamilton.

Christopher Robert Pemberton

Oils on canvas, 36 by 27¾ inches, by an unknown artist

Half length to right, writing, the head tilted to right and turned towards the spectator; close cut grey hair, touching collar, dark brown eyebrows, brown eyes, straight nose, clean shaven; white cravat, black coat; red curtain background. On the back modern labels giving the sitter's identity.

This, and the portrait of Mrs. Pemberton, were purchased from Mrs. Pemberton Cotton, July 1964.

The only published type is the portrait by Sir Thomas Lawrence *c.* 1810, which was *c.* 1964 in the collection of Stanley M. Pemberton of Washington, Sussex. Its dimensions are approximately the same as our portrait, which seems to be an early copy of it.

Ref: 'A Catalogue of the Paintings ... of Sir Thomas Lawrence' by K. Garlick, *Walpole Society*, XXXIX, 1964, p. 160; *Annals*, 30 July 1964, p. 229; information K. Garlick, Esq.

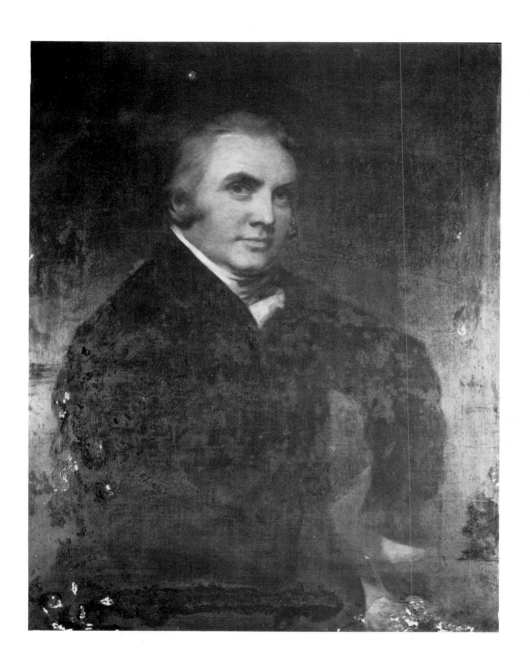

167

Sarah Pemberton

Oils on canvas, 30 by 25 inches, by an unknown artist

Head and shoulders, hands not shown; curly chestnut hair resting on shoulders, high arched dark brown eyebrows, large blue eyes, plump face, high colour; light v-necked lemon slip edged with white lace, roses in bosom, pale blue low-cut dress; plain background, lit from right. Stamp on the back of canvas: *JOHN – | ARTIST COLORMAN | JOHN ST | TOTTENHAM COURT RD*; also two modern labels identifying the sitter.

This, and the portrait of Christopher Robert Pemberton, were purchased from Mrs. Pemberton Cotton, July 1964.

Although having the same provenance as that of her husband, the portrait of Mrs. Pemberton does not derive from Lawrence but is by a lesser hand.

168

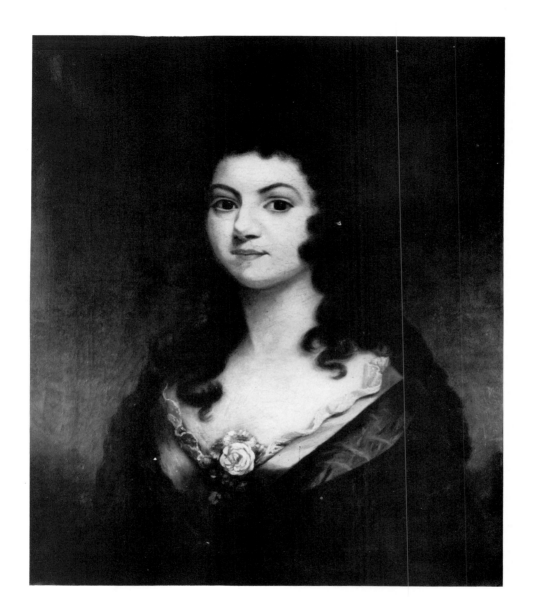

169

David Pitcairn 1749–1809 F. 1785

Son of a Scottish army officer who was killed at Bunker Hill, David Pitcairn became physician to St. Bartholomew's Hospital. He was a doctor whom other doctors consulted, and whose patients enjoyed his full care and attention, often without charge.

(Catalogue I, pp. 332–333)

2. Miniature, enamel, 4¾ by 3¾ inches (sight), by Henry Bone c. 1809, after John Hoppner

To waist, seated to left, hands not seen; curly white hair brushed back on top of forehead and covering the tip of ear, brown eyebrows, blue eyes looking at spectator, large nose, fresh complexion; white shirt ruffle, double-breasted brown velvet coat unbuttoned at waist, grey waistcoat; green upholstered chair, buttoned along top edge, plain brown background; lit from right. Inscribed in the same hands as on the back of the Bone of Matthew Baillie, and framed as a companion. The ink inscription on the backing paper reads: *David Pitcairn M.D. | Born 1749 | Died April 1809 |* , and in another hand *Pd. for the Enamel 45 | guineas | Frame 7. guineas |* , in another, *Henry Bone | 15 Berners Street* and another *From a Picture of Hoppner.*

Presented by Miss Angela Oliver, 1972.

Copied from the College's portrait, painted about 1800. Bone's reduced squared drawing in the National Portrait Gallery library is inscribed: *The late Dʳ. Pitcairn after Hoppner | for Mrs Baillie May 1809.*

Ref: Henry Bone, *Sketchbooks*, III, p. 13, N.P.G. library; *Catalogue*, I, 1964, pp. 332–333; *Annals*, 27 April 1972, p. 90a.

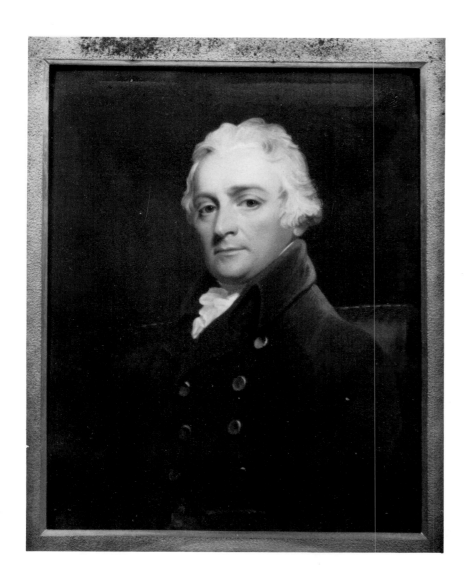

Robert Platt, 1st Baron Platt of Grindleford 1900– F. 1935 P. 1957–62

Born in London, Robert Platt qualified in medicine at Sheffield University Medical School. He was appointed physician to the Royal Infirmary, Sheffield; then from 1946–65 Professor of Medicine, Manchester University. A musician, he plays the cello in string quartets at the houses of friends, and was on various committees connected with music. During the second World War he served as consulting physician to the southern army in India and held the rank of brigadier. For ten years from 1948 he edited the *Quarterly Journal of Medicine*, He has been widely recognized as an authority on renal disease, hypertension and medical genetics.

Platt was elected President of the RCP in 1957 – the first 'provincial' to hold the office, which he filled for 5 years. In 1959 he was made a baronet, and created a Life Peer in 1967, in which year he gave the Harveian Oration. He played a leading role in the move of the College from Pall Mall East.

In 1957 he was Chairman of the Committee for Research in General Practice, and he also chaired a committee which reviewed the establishment of hospitals in the National Health Service (NHS), resulting in the Platt Report.

Platt has had a running battle with the BMA. In 1948 he resigned his membership because he disliked the Association's antagonism towards the NHS and, in 1963, when delivering the Rock Carling Lecture, he criticized the BMA for descending to the level of a trades union. During this lecture he also called for the reform of hospital management committees and boards of governors, etc., which he considered carried too high a proportion of 'relatively inefficient and inexpert onlookers'. Again in 1966 he was criticizing the BMA for its tactics; he accused it of making an enemy of the Ministry and felt that it had damaged the image of general practice in this country.

Platt has always cared greatly about the general practitioner, for whom he has a high regard, although he strongly disapproves of doctors who talk of strike action – which he regards as unforgivable in a professional man – and those who threaten to emigrate. He has suggested longer postgraduate training for potential GPs and at one time a system of financial rewards for doctors of outstanding ability.

Platt is also very concerned about the patient, whom he wants treated as an individual – to him there are no bad patients, only some who present more of a challenge than others. He considers there is a great need for better psychology in doctor-patient relations.

In 1962 the RCP report, *Smoking and Health*, was published; Lord Platt had chaired the Committee which had undertaken to examine smoking in relation to lung cancer and other diseases.

Platt has approved euthanasia in principle and, it seems, has had liberal views on abortion, although, as President of the Family Planning Association, he saw no need for the distribution of pamphlets on birth control in schools (contending that the types most likely to need such advice were the ones least likely to seek or accept it).

Retired now and living in Esher, but active in the House of Lords and still making music with and for his friends. He has written an autobiography, *Private and Controversial*, published in 1972.

Lord Platt]

Oils on canvas, 49 ½ by 39 ½ inches, by Merlyn Evans, 1963

Nearly whole length, seated to left, hands on arms of wooden chair; smooth dark grey hair, parted on left, dark grey eyebrows, brown eyes, thin upper lip; white collar and shirt, black tie, plain dark grey coat and trousers; light brown background, suggesting an interior wall; lit from the right. Signed in red, bottom left: *Evans, 63*.

Commissioned by the College.

A photograph was taken for the National Photographic Record in 1959.

174   *Ref: Annals*, 25 April 1963, p. 73.

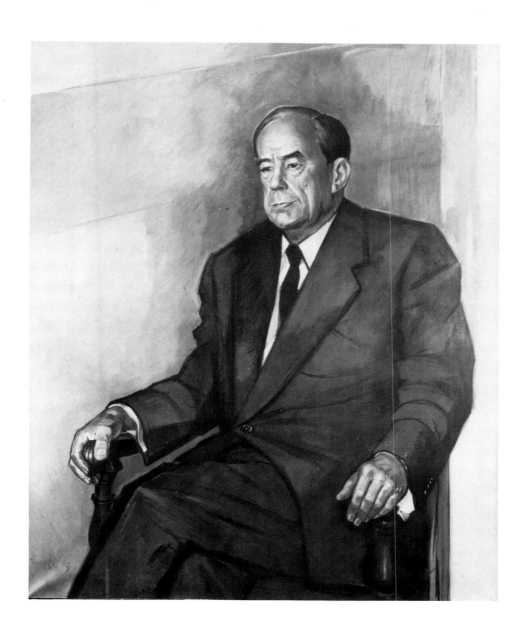

Clive Riviere 1872–1929 F. 1909

Born in Gloucestershire, the son of a Royal Academician. He began his education at St Andrew's University; then at University College School and University College, London, before studying medicine at Barts and Tübingen University.

At Barts., his interest in diseases of the chest began. When he died he was physician to the City of London Hospital for Diseases of the Chest and here he had gained his worldwide reputation. As a pioneer in artificial pneumothorax treatment, he was renowned for his extraordinarily light touch and is said to have had a 'well-nigh perfect technique'.

His three publications, *Tuberculin Treatment* (1912, in collaboration with E.C. Morland), *The Early Diagnosis of Tubercle* (1914) and *The Pneumothorax Treatment of Tuberculosis* (1917) illustrate best where his special interests and talents lay.

A man of charm and transparent integrity; sensitive to suffering; liked music, reading, the countryside; modest; never in the least petty or jealous, he stayed away from professional politics, whilst achieving a reputation for success in organizing international congresses.

Pneumonia killed him after a week's illness.

Oils on paper, 10 by 12 inches, by himself, 1925

Head and shoulders, full face, wearing spectacles; grey hair. Inscribed (probably by the artist) in pencil on the back: *At Menaggio (Como) Mar 1925 Self Portrait C Riviere.*

176   *Ref:* Catalogue I, 1964, p. 455.

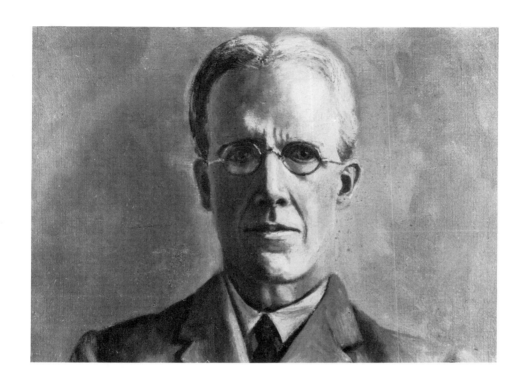

Sir Kenneth Robson 1909- F. 1943

Kenneth Robson was educated at Bradfield School, Christ's College, Cambridge, and the Middlesex Hospital where he qualified in 1933.

In 1938 he was appointed physician to St George's Hospital but from 1939–1946 he served in the Royal Air Force, in charge of medical divisions of hospitals in England and India, ending the war as Air Commodore and Consultant in Medicine to the RAF in India and the Far East. Since 1949 he has been Civil Consultant-in-Medicine to the RAF.

Kenneth Robson's main interest has been in diseases of the chest. He was secretary of the Thoracic Society from 1947–60, and its President in 1965.

For the RCP Kenneth Robson has served as examiner, Censor, Goulstonian Lecturer, and from 1961–1975 as an outstanding Registrar. Unmarried, he devoted much of his life to every aspect of the welfare of the College. He was created CBE in 1959 and knighted in 1968.

Oils on canvas, 36 by 27¾ inches, by Walter Woodington, 1975

Three-quarter length seated and looking to right, elbows resting on arms of chair, hands clasped in lap; receding grey hair, grey(?) eyes and eyebrows; Cambridge M.D. gown over plain dark blue lounge suit, light blue soft shirt, plain dark blue tie; wooden chair, light blue background. Signed and dated bottom left: *Woodington 1975.*

Commissioned by the College, 1975.

A photograph for the National Photographic Record was taken in 1970.

178   *Ref:* R.A. catalogue 1975 (924); *Annals*, 31 July 1975, Doc. 13.

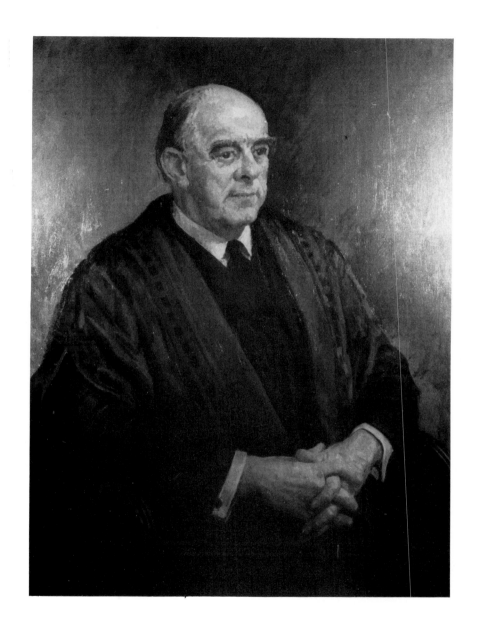

179

Max Leonard Rosenheim, 1st Baron Rosenheim of Camden 1908–1972 F. 1941 P. 1966–1972

Born in London, and educated at Shrewsbury School; St John's College, Cambridge; and University College Hospital Medical School.

In 1938 he was awarded the Bilton Pollard Travelling Fellowship and worked as research assistant for Dr Fuller Albright at the Massachusetts General Hospital. On his return from Boston, he worked with Professor (later, Sir) Harold Himsworth.

He joined the RAMC in 1941 and served in the Middle East and Italy. He left the Army as a brigadier, though nobody looked less like a military man than he did. In 1945–46, Rosenheim was consultant physician to the Allied Land Forces in South East Asia, giving him a lifelong interest in medicine and medical education throughout that vast area. From 1949 for the next 21 years, he was Professor of Medicine at UCH, but resigned his Chair when he felt he could not devote enough time to it. He retained his links with UCH, however, acting as a part-time physician to the Hospital.

As the Sir Arthur Sims Commonwealth Travelling Professor in 1958, he visited Australia and New Zealand – and these commonwealth links were to be forged more strongly later on when he was President of the RCP, to which he was elected in 1966. Max Rosenheim was a great traveller and, under him, the College expanded its activities and its membership, and ceased to be merely a London club for physicians – a criticism that had been levelled at it in the past. Max Rosenheim was particularly concerned about postgraduate medical education, and medical education in developing countries. He also passionately wanted the general public to receive better health education. Other fervent concerns of his were cigarette-smoking, which he again and again called on the Government to ban; alcoholism; the need for fluoridation of drinking water; the quality of life. He spoke often about the old and it obviously worried him that, although it was now possible to prolong life, the quality of that life was not necessarily good, and he questioned the amount of money spent on research, wondering whether we had not reached a point when we might devote ourselves more to the application of the knowledge already gained than spend large sums on increasing our knowledge still further.

In 1972 he was admitted FRS by special election. His own particular medical interests were renal disease and hypertension, and he was among the first in his profession to convince his fellows that hypertension could be treated. A large proportion of his patients were themselves doctors and their relatives.

He never married, but was a devoted son of a mother who died only shortly before he did. Friends said that he 'suffered fools gladly'. A stout, genial figure, comfortable to be with, he needed only five hours' sleep and had time for all those who sought his advice; an excellent mediator, Max was very good at getting people to co-operate, and is remembered with real affection by a host of colleagues and patients.

Lord Rosenheim]

Lord Rosenheim]

1. Oil (acrylic(?)) on canvas, 36¼ by 28¼ inches, by Judy Cassab, 1972

Half length to left, seated in wooden chair, his right hand and left forearm on the chair arms; greying hair brushed close, eyes looking at spectator, light eyebrows, brown spectacles, dimpled chin; soft white shirt, plain blue tie, plain blue lounge suit, the coat fastened with single button, blue background, lighter behind head. Signed bottom right: *Cassab / 1972*.

Commissioned by the College; received 1973. Exhibited at the Royal Academy 1973, their label on back.

Ref: Annals, 25 January 1973, p. 32.

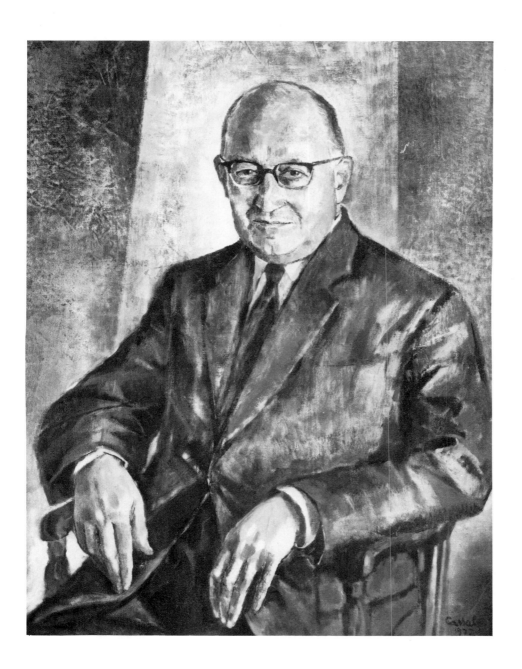

183

Lord Rosenheim]

2. *Oil (acrylic(?)) on canvas, 20 by 16 inches, by Rhoda Pepys*

Head and shoulders, looking to right; receding grey hair, spectacles, double chin, eyes and right side of face in green shadow, yellow flesh colour, pink shirt, purple tie, light blue coat; scarlet background shading to purple at edges. Signed, bottom right: *RHODA | PEPYS.* Inscribed in black on the back of the canvas: *163 | PROFESSOR | SIR MAX ROSENHEIM | By Rhoda Pepys | London 1966.*

Presented by the artist, 1973.

3. *Brown chalk on buff(?) paper, 17 by 11½ inches, by Rhoda Pepys (not reproduced here)*

Head only, sketch for the above; signed *Pepys* bottom right. Inscribed on the back: *No. 7. | Professor Sir Max Rosenheim | P.R.C.P. | By Rhoda Pepys.*

Presented by the artist, 1973.

A photograph was taken for the National Photographic Record in 1969 by Lotte Meitner-Graf.

184   *Ref:* al. from J. Pepys (undated) and from the Registrar 19 June 1973.

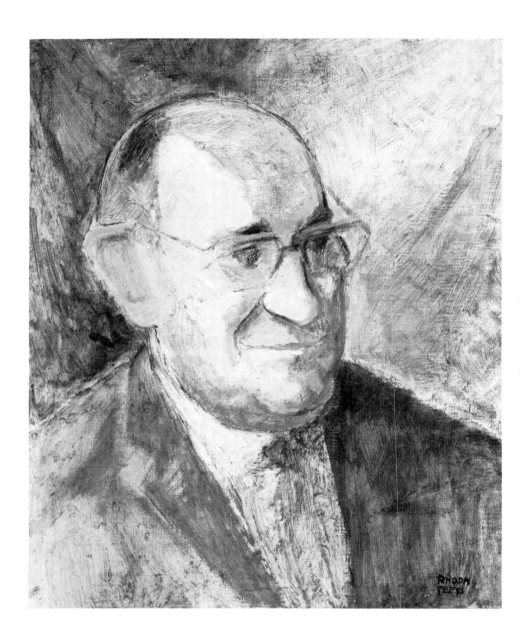

185

Albert Schweitzer 1875–1965

Musician, philosopher, theologian, author and physician, Albert Schweitzer, like all extraordinary individuals, has been, and still is, the subject of heated controversy. Those for him and those against him tend to adopt extreme attitudes, and Schweitzer is either loved and revered as a saint or denounced as an egoist and even, by some as a rogue.

Born in Kayserberg, Alsace, 14 January 1875 into a musical and devout family – his father was pastor of Kayserberg – the combined atmosphere of religion and music in which Albert grew up was to determine the pattern of his career. He began playing the organ at eight and deputized for the local church organist by the time he was nine. Surprisingly, ordinary schoolwork was harder for him to master.

In 1912 he married Helene Bresslau and, a year later, he and his wife set out for Lambaréné in French Equatorial Africa where, at Schweitzer's own expense, he built his famous hospital. For the rest of his life he was to commute between Africa and Europe, raising funds by giving lectures and organ recitals.

Schweitzer has been called paternalistic and authoritarian; he demanded of one of his colleagues that Lambaréné be regarded as Mount Olympus, and himself as Zeus. His rages were formidable but soon over. Critics have cast doubt on the quality of the medicine practised at the hospital. Certainly Lambaréné was run on un-orthodox lines: patients were permitted to surround themselves with their relatives and pets – a concession that had the virtue of making them feel more at home and less afraid of the white man's mysterious medicine.

Schweitzer was awarded the Nobel Peace Prize in 1952 and the Order of Merit in 1955.

He died, a very old and much honoured man, at his beloved Lambaréné. His wife had predeceased him; they had one daughter.

Oils on canvas, 35¾ by 28 inches, by Felix Szezesny Kwarta, 1953

Three-quarter length to right, standing in a landscape, head bent forward, hands clasped round book; bushy grey hair, grey eyebrows, dark brown eyes, bushy grey moustache covering upper lip, sun tanned complexion; white bush(?) jacket, open at neck; river landscape with mountains on low horizon, cloudy sky dark grey at top of picture with ray of sun on right. Signed in red up the right hand edge: *f.s. kwarta*.

Presented by Mrs. C. Pugh, October 1967.

Presumably the portrait exhibited at the Royal Society of Portrait Painters 1953 (159); reproduced in *The Times*, 20 November 1953. On the back a label from the R.S.P.P. exhibition. The background indicates the sitter's native Rhineland. Other portraits include a painting by Clara Ewald; busts by Louise Hutchinson, exhibited Society of Portrait Sculptors 1956 (52) and L. Cubitt Bevis, Royal Academy 1963 (1240) and H. B. Huxley-Jones, Society of Portrait Sculptors 1966 (9); and, among photographs, the well known example by Yousuf Karsh 1954.

Ref: *The Times*, 20 November 1953; R.S.P.P. catalogue 1956; Y. Karsh, *Portraits of Greatness*, 1959, p. 178; R.A. catalogue 1963; S.P.S. catalogue 1966; *Annals*, 26 October 1967, p. 147; *Commentary*, July 1968, p. 82.

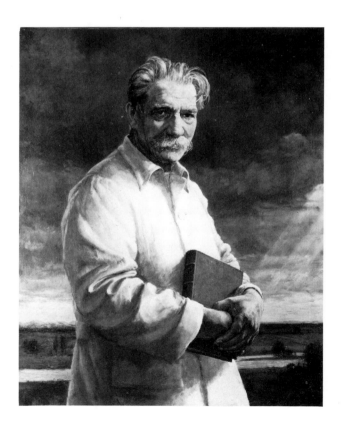

(?) Thomas Sydenham 1624–1689   L. 1663

Called 'the Father of English Medicine' and 'the English Hippocrates', Sydenham taught the value of clinical observation and the importance of allowing nature to effect a cure. He revolutionized the care of fevers, identified hysteria, discovered convulsions in childhood (Sydenham's chorea), and became a sufferer from and authority on gout. Friend of Robert Boyle and John Locke, and revered in Europe.

(Catalogue I, pp. 396–405)

5. Oils on canvas, 24 ¼ by 20 inches, by an unknown artist

Short half length to right, hands not shewn; dark brown wig, resting on shoulders, dark brown eyebrows, dark brown eyes, straight nose, heavy jowl, cleanshaven; white shirt and necktie, brown lace cravat, brown gown, with a suggestion of gold lace; dark background. On the centre bar of the stretcher, in a late eighteenth(?) century hand, in black paint: *Portrait of Dr Tho[s] Sydenham | by | Mrs Beale.;* on the bottom bar a cutting from p. 13 of a printed catalogue *BEALE, MARY (1632–1697) | 254 Portrait of Dr. Thomas Sydenham (circa 1685–90) in costume of the period, with dark, | flowing wig. 22 ½ in. by 19., in gilt frame.*

Presented by Dr. Bruce Maclean, F.R.C.P., January 1965.

It is not certain that the brading on the gown is authentic; there is no conspicuously additional paint, which runs over the craquelure, but on the other hand the pigment here does not look contemporary. Though worn, there remain passages of greater distinction than is normally found in the work of Mary Beale, as in, for example, the cravat; and it may be that the attribution as well as the identification is comparatively modern. The provenance has not been traced and identification rests on comparison with authentic portraits. That of Thomas Sydenham by Mary Beale painted in 1688 in the National Portrait Gallery shews a man of quite other mien, as does the different type presented to the College (2) by the sitter's son in 1691. There is a slightly closer resemblance to the oval portrait in the College (3), but this is itself a derivation of the Beale type, probably through Blooteling's engraving, and the sitter in (5) looks too young for Sydenham. The portrait is not closely datable, but must be post 1660, and perhaps as late as *c.* 1680. If a member of the Sydenham family, the likeliest candidate would be one of Thomas Sydenham's three sons, William Sydenham, L.R.C.P., pensioner of Pembroke *c.* 1674, *d.c.* 1738, but no portraits are known for comparison.

Ref: G. F. Sydenham, *The History of the Sydenham Family*, privately printed, 1928; *Catalogue,* 1964, pp. 396–405; *Annals,* 28 January 1965, p. 5.

188

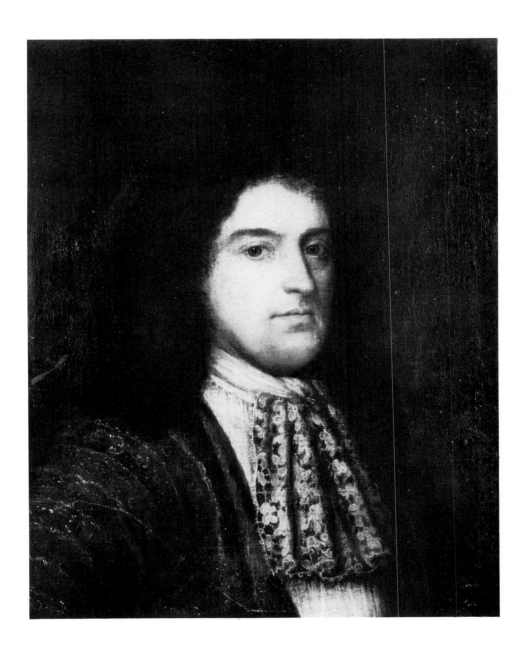

189

Unknown man by Richmond

Drawing, black chalk, heightened with white, on paper originally white, 24 by 18 inches, by George Richmond, 1856

Head and shoulders to left, head tilted slightly forward and eyes looking at spectator, the left shoulder cut by the picture edge, the hands not shewn; very dark brown wavy hair, side whiskers, point of chin clean shaven, thick eyebrows, narrow lips touched with carmine; tall shirt collar, coat and waistcoat lightly indicated. Signed and dated, bottom left: *George Richmond delit. 1856.* Laid down on a cardboard mount 25¾ by 19¾ inches. As with many of Richmond's drawings, the colour of the paper has changed to mid-brown, leaving the work now very much out of key.

Source and date of acquisition unknown.

The sitter is not Dr. P. M. Latham, the copyright of which is entered in Richmond's accounts for 1854. Richmond's drawing of him, an older man, looking to the right, was engraved by F. Holl. It has not proved possible to equate our drawing with any of the extracts *c.* 1856 from Richmond's diaries, a copy of which is in the library of the National Portrait Gallery.

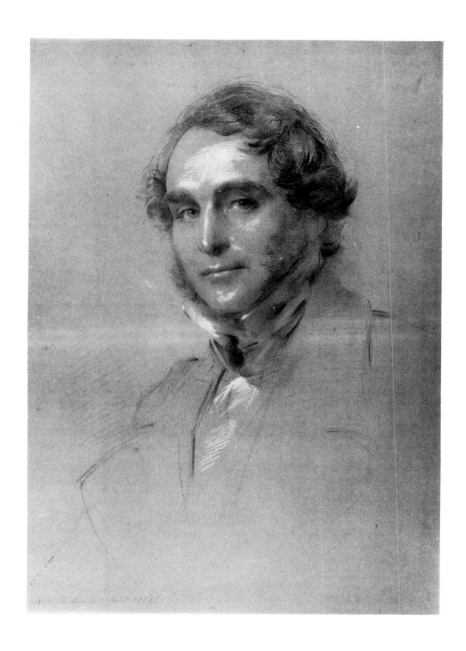

191

Anne (Lady) Whitmore d. 1775

Wife of Sir Thomas Whitmore KB.

Oils on canvas, 50⅜ by 40⅛ inches, by Edward Penny, 1757

Nearly whole length, seated to left, but looking towards spectator, her right wrist on table her left hand in lap; dark brown eyebrows, blue eyes, dark brown hair dressed with pearls, short lips, fresh complexion; golden half-sleeved dress with white lace collar and cuffs, two rows of pearls at bosom and four on her left wrist; tall blue-upholstered chair, blue curtain and tassel on left, plain background. Signed, or inscribed, and dated bottom left: *E.Penney Pinx. 1757.*

Inscribed top right, the inscription now rather illegible:
Ann[e?] Wife to Sʳ Tho. Whitmore/Eldest Daughter to Sʳ Jonathan Cope Bart. / AEtalis Suae 39 E Penn[e?]y pinx 17 [57?]

Property of the Harveian Society of London, lent to the College November 1968.

Anonymous property, Christies 11 December 1964, lot 53, bt. Agnew, as Anne, wife of Sir Thomas Whitmore, K.B., daughter of Sir Jonathan Cope of Brewern, aged 39. A portrait of Sir Thomas's sister Catherine, also by Penny (misread Penner in the sale catalogue) was the previous lot. The portraits of Sir Eliab and Lady Harvey, *above*, also bought Agnew, were lot 54 of the sale.

Ref: Correspondence, Harveian Society 1 and 6 November 1968.

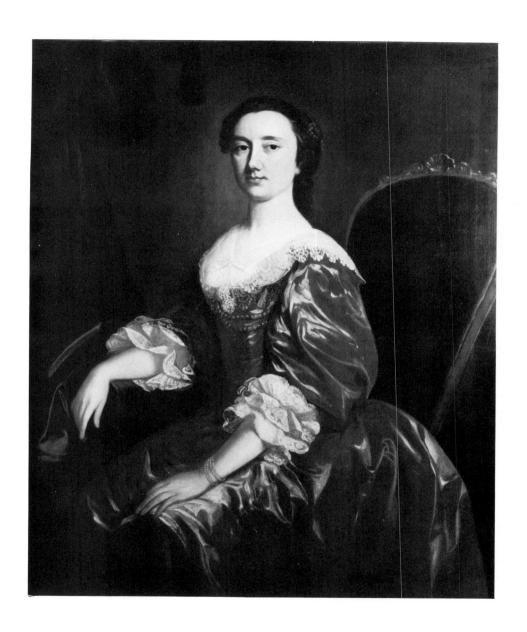

193

Sir William James Erasmus Wilson 1809–84

Known as Erasmus Wilson, he was born in Marylebone, London.

In 1836 he established Sydenham College, a school of anatomy, which, however, failed. He was himself a skilful draughtsman and his anatomical sketches were very fine. On the advice of a colleague, sometime around 1840, he switched from anatomy and physiology to dermatology. Dermatology was then a virtually untried area of medicine. Erasmus was to become extremely successful and the money he made he invested cleverly so that he ended up a very rich man – he left some £200,000 at his death. It is said that he knew more about diseases of the skin than any of his contemporaries. To broaden his knowledge on the subject, he travelled extensively, as far as Ethiopia.

There are three outstanding things, among many, that he did with his money: (1) he founded in 1870 a Chair of Dermatology at the Royal College of Surgeons, which he was the first to occupy; (2) he paid some £10,000 for the transportation of Cleopatra's Needle to London in 1877; and (3) he established the Erasmus Wilson Professorship of Pathology at Aberdeen University in 1881 in his father's memory. He was clearly an unusually generous man and his benefactions were numerous and varied.

Wilson became a Fellow of the Royal College of Surgeons in 1843 and in 1881 was elected President. The RCS benefited substantially from his generosity: not only did he establish the Chair of Dermatology and, in addition, donate his collection of anatomical specimens, drawings, etc., but the bulk of his fortune went to the College after his wife's death; (they had no children).

In 1857 he saved the life of a would-be suicide who tried to drown herself and was awarded the Royal Humane Society's silver medal.

To Erasmus Wilson is given the credit for popularizing the bath among the middle- and upper-classes!

At one stage in his career, he was asked to give evidence in the case of a man who had apparently died from the injuries inflicted by a regimental flogging. Wilson confirmed that this was the cause of the man's death and, after ten adjournments, the jury supported him by bringing in a verdict to that effect. A Parliamentary enquiry followed and this in turn led to the abolition of flogging in the army.

Oils on canvas, now 30 by 25 inches, (?) by Stephen Pearce of c. 1872

Short half length to left, head turned towards spectator; curly grey hair and side whiskers, grey eyebrows, blue eyes, fresh complexion; white collar and shirt, loosely tied black bow, black coat, black gown with crimson edges; a beige-covered table(?) bottom left; plain brown background, a window extreme left; lit from the right.

Property of the British Association of Dermatology, on loan to the College July 1963.

Pearce wrote that he painted three portraits of Wilson in his robes as Professor of Dermatology. The sitter was an old friend whom he had known since 1852 or 3. He exhibited one at the R.A. in 1873. Three versions are known at present: that in the Middlesex Hospital; that on loan to the College, which measured 50 by 40 inches when in the London art trade in 1962 before its purchase by the British Association of Dermatology; and a copy by John Lewis Reilly, also 50 by 40 inches, presented to the Royal College of Surgeons of England in 1898. An engraving of the type by Alexander Scott, R.A., 1873 (1302) was published by Graves in 1873. Wilson was also painted by J. Andrews R.A., 1854 (1129). A marble bust by Thomas Brock was commissioned by the Royal College of Surgeons, May 1885 and completed 1888. Brock also was responsible for the bronze statue erected in front of the Margate Infirmary 1886, of which, like the Royal College of Surgeons of England, the sitter had been a benefactor.

Ref: R.A. catalogues 1854 (1129); 1872 (431); 1873 (1302); 1885 (2042, an unidentified marble); 1886 (1772, the Margate bronze); 1888 (1969, the R.C.S. marble); S. Pearce, *Memories of the Past*, 1903, pp. 85–87; W. LeFanu, 1960, p. 76; al. from the British Association of Dermatology, 6 July 1963.

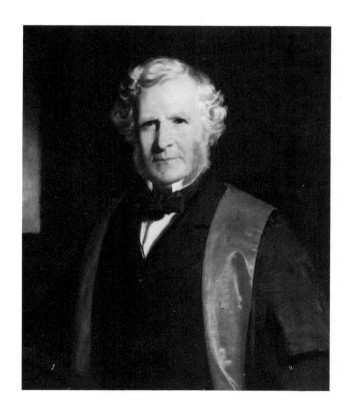

Sir Isaac Wolfson Bt. 1897–   Hon. F. 1959

The young Wolfson left Queens Park School, Glasgow, at the age of 14 and worked in his father's cabinet-making business in Glasgow, earning 5 shillings a week. His father was a refugee from East Europe. When Isaac was only 9 his father referred to him as 'a financial genius'.

In his 20's, Isaac Wolfson went to London, starting as supplier and merchandise consultant to Great Universal Stores (GUS – the mail order business), becoming joint Managing Director, with Mr George Rose, in 1932, and Chairman in 1946. Under his guidance, GUS pioneered the mass production of furniture. An article in the *Sunday Times* (1961) called him 'one of the greatest shopkeepers in this nation of shopkeepers'.

In 1955 he founded and became Trustee and first Chairman of the Wolfson Foundation for the advancement of health, education and youth activities in the UK and Commonwealth. A magnificent donation from the Foundation to the RCP, through the mediation of Lord Evans (q.v.), largely made possible the move of the College to its splendid premises in Regent's Park.

Deeply religious, Wolfson is devoted to Israel, where he is a Trustee of the Religious Centre in Jerusalem and Honorary President and Fellow of the Weizmann Institute of Science.

An emotional, volatile man with great warmth and charm; non-smoker and tee-totaller; an enthusiast, always teeming with ideas; at times undeniably demanding of others but totally commanding their loyalty. Thickset and handsome, the *Sunday Times* described him as 'Spencer Tracy playing the part of Isaac Wolfson'.

Bronze bust, 22 inches high, including base 2 ¼ inches high, by Sir William Reid Dick, 1953

Head and shoulders, slightly receding hair brushed back, eyes directed slightly to right, lips parted; coat with broad lapels, waistcoat, soft collar, tie; incised on the back of the shoulders: *W REID DICK 53.*

Commissioned by the College, 1966.

A replica made by the Art Bronze Foundry of the original in the sitter's possession, which was presumably the bust exhibited at the Royal Academy, 1954 (1236); the sitter was painted by Sir James Gunn, Royal Academy, 1955 (303). A photograph was taken by Godfrey Argent for the National Photographic Record in 1969.

Ref: Royal Academy Illustrated, 1954, p. 87; *Commentary*, July 1968, p. 81.

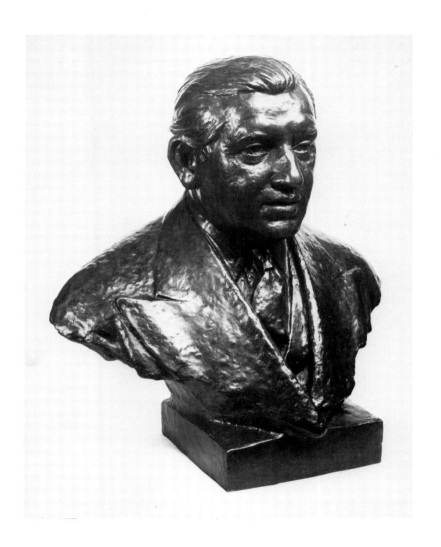

The medals

Sir William Browne 1692–1774
F. 1726 P. 1765–66

(Catalogue I, pp. 92–93)

2. By William Wyon, gold, 1 7/16 inches diameter

Obverse. Head and shoulders portrait of Browne, profile to left, in wig, bands and President's (?) gown; *D GVILELMVS BROWNE EQVES. | NAT. III. NON* (sic) *. IAN. A. | MDCXCII* below and *ESSE ET VIDERI* around bust; i.e. as described save that our specimens have *NON* in error for *NOV*.

Reverse. *SVNT SVA PRAEMIA LAVDI.* Apollo, seated on a plinth with lyre, extends wreath to kneeling student; below *ELECTVS COLL. MED. | LOND. PRAESES.A.S. | MDCCLXV.*; suspensory frame inscribed *H.H.KNAPP LATIN ODE 1803.*

From the collection of H. H. Knapp, as incised.

Ref: Storer (500); Freeman (82).

3–4. Two silver strikes, as above

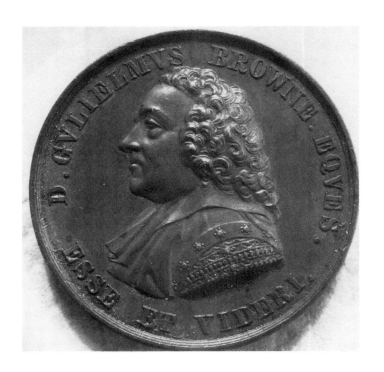

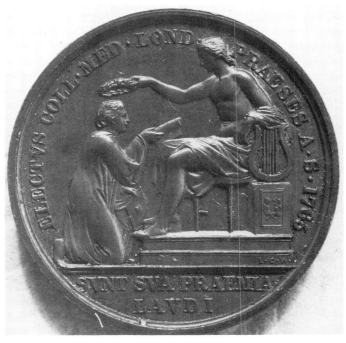

Sir William Browne]

5. *Bronze, 1 inch diameter*

Obverse as above.

Reverse by Leonard Charles Wyon. Same design as 2–4, but the figures of Apollo and the student more neoclassical in style and appear younger; the lettering is juxtaposed, the line *SVNT* etc. being placed below; signed with initials *L.C.W.* on the plinth.

Prize medal for Greek and Latin odes and epigrams at Cambridge.

202   *Ref:* Forrer, VI, p. 628; *Catalogue*, I, 1964, pp. 92–93.

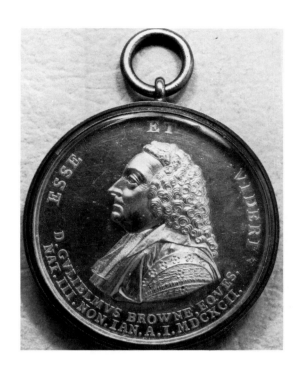

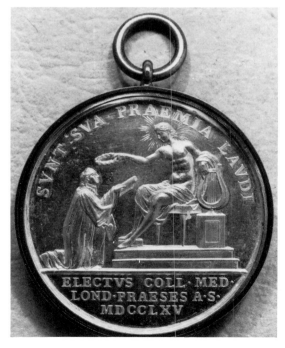

203

John Freind 1675–1728 F. 1716

(Catalogue I, 170–173; catalogue II, 108–109)

4. Not located in 1963, but then thought likely to be a strike of the bronze medallion by Ferdinand de St. Urbain

Bust inscribed *IOANNES.FREIND.COLL..MED.LOND.ET.REG.S.S.* and, on the truncation, *S V* (the artist's monogram, for St. Urbain). On the reverse, an ancient and modern physician shake hands: inscribed *MEDICINA VETVS ET NOVA*, and, *VNAM FACIMVS VTRAMQVE*, and again the signature *S V*. (Based on Hawkin's description of St. Urbain's medal.).

Presented in 1879 by the Reverend C. B. Norcliffe of York.

The allusion appears to be to Freind's *History of Physic*, published in 1726, which advocates a synthesis of old and new practice in medicine. The medal may be posthumous.

Ref: Annals, 9 May 1879; Hawkins, II, 1885, p. 488; Forrer, V, 1912, p. 311 (reproduction).

4. Medal by Ferdinand St. Urbain, bronze, 2 ⅛ inches (54 mm.) diameter

This medal has now been found and is as described above.

204   *Ref: Catalogue* I, 1964, p. 172.

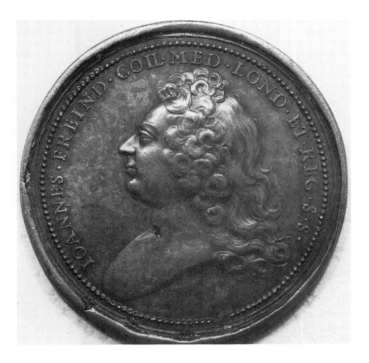

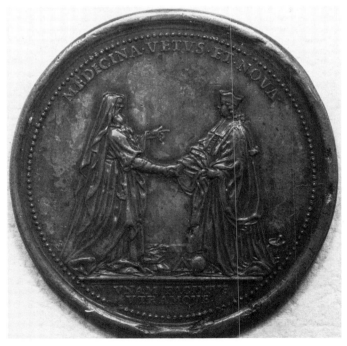

205

Thomas Guy 1645(?)–1724

After (?) Leonard Charles Wyon, gold(?), 1¹⁵⁄₁₆ inches (48.5 mm.) diameter

Obverse: laureated shield of arms of Guy's Hospital above the motto *DARE QUAM ACCIPERE;* letters inside the rim RICHARD BRIGHT 1827 · GUY'S HOSPITAL · 1927.

Reverse: Seen through a 'window' Thomas Guy receiving a male patient in the forecourt of the Hospital, both whole length; signed *WYON* on the exergue. The portrait is based on the monument of 1779 to Guy by John Bacon in the Hospital Chapel.

A reissue, with appropriate rewording on the obverse, of Wyon's design of the Guy's Hospital medal for Clinical Surgery.

Presented to [Sir] John Rose Bradford (8 July 1927) as incised.

Centenary of discovery of Bright's disease, 1927.

The obverse is a portrait based on the monument of 1779 to Guy by John Bacon, in the Hospital chapel; the reverse is a reuse of a design by L. C. Wyon.

Forrer, VI, p. 630; *Lancet*, 16 July 1927; H. A. Ripman, *Guy's Hospital 1725–1948*, 1951, front. and opp. p. 144.

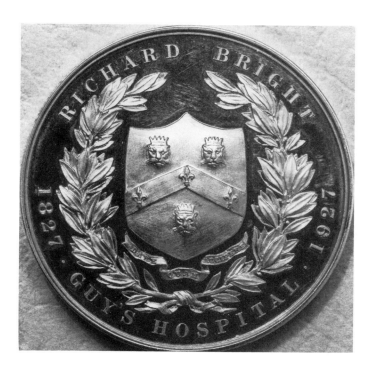

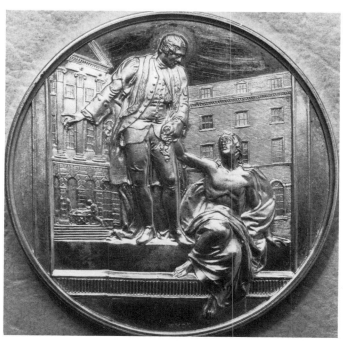

207

William Harvey 1578–1657 F. 1607

(Catalogue I, 202–215; catalogue II, 132–133)

7. By Charles Leonard Hartwell, bronze, 2 inches (51.5 mm.) diameter

Obverse. Head and shoulders of Harvey nearly profile to left, own hair, moustache and chin tuft; derives mainly from the College's bust by Scheemakers (Catalogue I, 210–11) lettered round the portrait, to left + *WILLIAM HARVEY* + and, to right, + *1578–1657* +; signed with initials below the cutaway *CLH.*

Reverse. Small profile of tonsured monk (Rahere), close-shaven, on plinth within an open laurel; lettered round within the rim + *1123* + *TO COMMEMORATE THE 800th ANNI-VERSARY* + *1923 St. BARTHOLOMEWS HOSPITAL* +; signed with initials below the bust *C.L.H.*

St. Bartholomew's Hospital Octocentenary 1923; commissioned by the Governors. 'Dr. William Harvey – medallion' which the artist exhibited at the Royal Academy 1923 (1370) was presumably a version of the College's medal.

Ref: R.A. catalogue 1923; *Catalogue* I, 1964, pp. 205–215; information from the Archivist, St. Bartholomew's Hospital, 1976.

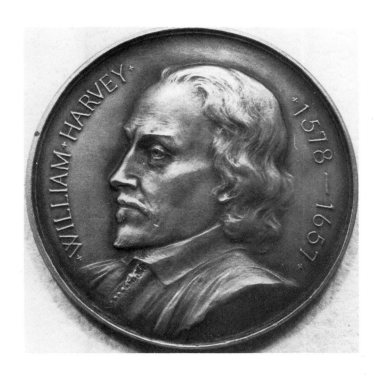

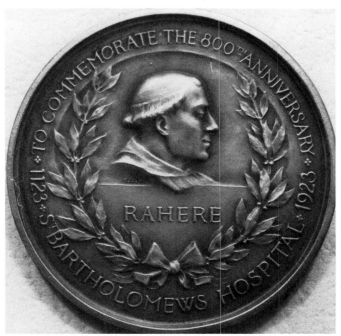

209

William Harvey]

8. By Charles d'O. Pilkington Jackson, 1923,? bronze, 1½ inches (38.5 mm.)

Obverse. Portrait of Harvey profile to left, deriving from the College's painting (Catalogue I, 204–05): lettered round the edge *WILLIAM* to left of portrait, *HARVEY* to right of it and *1578–1657* below; signed *PILKINGTON JACKSON* on the cutaway.

Reverse. Plain; lettered horizontally *INTER- | NATIONAL | PHYSIOLOGICAL | CON-GRESS —— | EDINBVRGH | 1923.*

Eleventh Physiological Congress, Edinburgh, 1923.

210   *Ref:* Freeman (763).

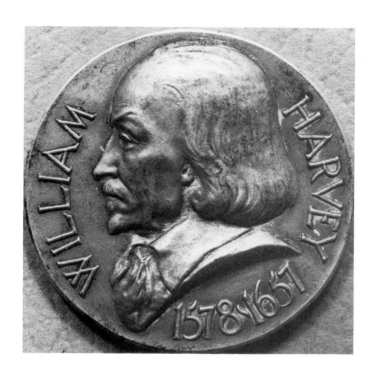

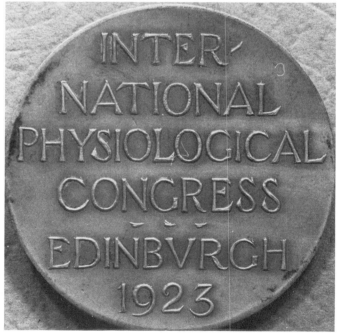

Alfredo Antunes Kanthack 1863–1898 F. 1897

By C. J. Allen, reverse by J. H. McNair, bronze, pointed oval 3¾ by 2⅝ inches (95 by 65 mm.)

Obverse. Bust of Kanthack, profile to left, hair brushed back behind ear, pince-nez, drooping moustache on upper lip, chin clean-shaven, wing collar and tie, laurel sprigs below; lettered round the bust: *PATHOLOGIST STVDENT OF VNIVERSITY COLL. LIVERPOOL* and below *ALFREDO | ANTVNES | KANTHACK 1863–1898;* signed by *C. J. ALLEN 190(0?)* below right hand twig.

Reverse. Beneath a nude female bust (?death) with crossed hands, a double panel enclosing twined branches; signed near bottom *1900 J. H. McNAIR.* Conferred by Thomson Yates laboratories upon students in experimental pathology; C. J. Allen exhibited the Kanthack Memorial medal at the R.A. 1901.

212   *Ref:* Forrer, I, p. 41; Storer (1865); R.A. catalogue 1901 (1746).

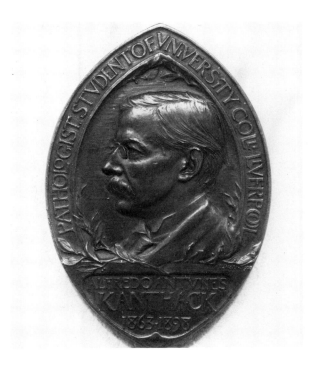

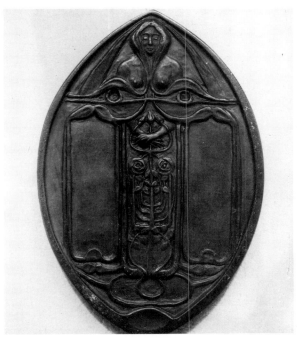

213

Charles Laubry 1872–1960 F. 1953

By P. M. Dammann, 1930, bronze, 3 1/16 inches (80 mm.) diameter

Obverse. Portrait of Laubry, profile to left, short hair with loose ends, spectacles, moustache on upper lip, pimple on cheek level with lower lip; stiff collar, gown; lettered to left: *CH – LAVBRY | MEDECIN DE L' HO | PITAL BROVSSAIS*, and to right, *P. M. DAMMANN | MCMXXX.*
Reverse blank.

Presumably by Paul Marcel Dammann, one of the sitter's patients.

Given by Dr. Evan Bedford, 1973.

214   *Ref:* Forrer, VII, p. 202; RCP Library Committee. *Minutes,* 2 January 1974, Doc. 5.

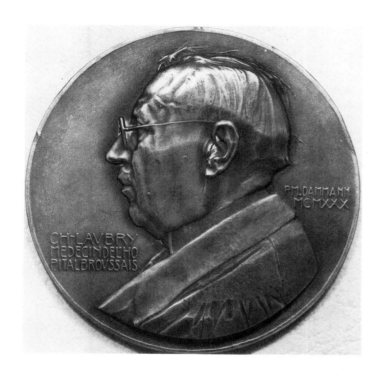

215

Richard Mead 1673–1754 F. 1716

(Catalogue I, pp. 282–291)

7. Medal by Leonard Charles Wyon and Allan Wyon, silver (?), 2⅞ inches (73 mm.) diameter

Obverse. Togated portrait in profile to right (based on the bust by Roubiliac, *Catalogue* I, 1964, pp. 290–91), own hair; lettered vertically *RICHARD MEAD M.D.* and signed below *L. C. WYON. SC.*

Reverse. Medical student seated, whole length to right in laboratory; he holds a specimen; on left A. WYON; shield of arms; lettered below a double rule *ST THOMAS'S | HOSPITAL.*

Given by Dr. A. M. Cooke, 1974.

A medical prize established in 1874.

Ref: Storer (2408), with different reverse; Forrer, VI, p. 629; *Catalogue* I, 1964, pp. 282–291; RCP Library Committee. *Minutes*, 3 July 1974, Doc. 13.

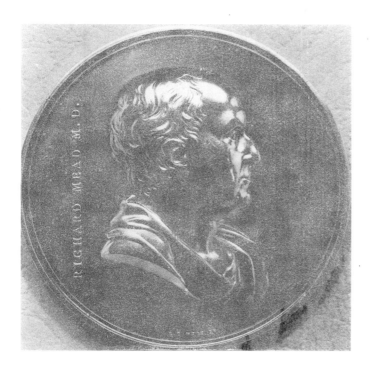

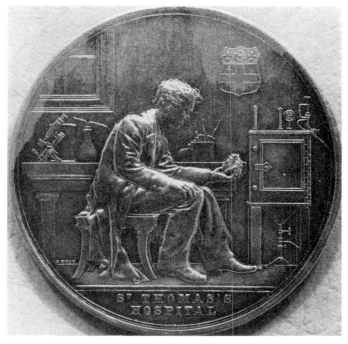

217

Sir William Osler, Bt. 1849–1919 F. 1883

(Catalogue I, pp. 320–321)

2. By Frank Bowcher [1925], bronze, 2⅞ inches (65 mm.) diameter

Obverse. Profile portrait of Osler to right, slightly receding hair cut short, curling moustache on upper lip, the chin clean-shaven; tall collar, plain coat; lettered round the circumference: *WILLEMUS OSLER, MEDICINAE PROFESSOR REGIUS MCMIV–XIX*; signed below the cutaway *F.B.*

Reverse. The circumference lettered *DE AESCULAPIO ARTE VEL SCIENTIA EXIMIE MERITUS.*, the arms of Oxford University within; signed below *F, BOWCHER, F.*

Oxford University medical prize, first awarded 1925, thereafter quinquennially. The portrait is based on the plaque by Frédéric Charles Victor de Vernon, Paris, 1903, Freeman (374).

218   *Ref:* Storer (2662a); Freeman (377); *Catalogue* I, 1964, p. 320.

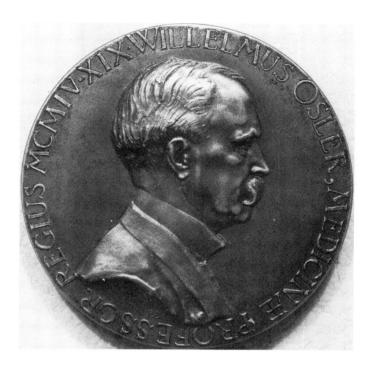

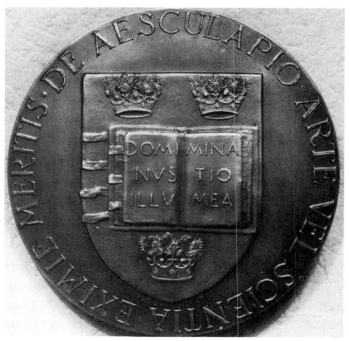

Edouard Rist 1871–1956 F. 1940

By P. M. Dammann [1950], bronze, 3 1/16 inches (80 mm.) diameter

Obverse. Profile portrait of Rist to left, smooth receding hair, spectacles, moustache on upper lip, coat, collar and tie; *EDOVARD RIST* on either side of head, *P. M. DAMMANN* below.

Reverse. A nude nymph seated to right, on a monster, offers fruit to a rayed sun, cloud on left (knowledge overcoming ignorance?); below *FERVIDO LVCEM | QVAESIT ANIMO.*

Presented by Dr. R. Hilton.

220   *Ref: Annals,* 30 January 1964, p. 145.

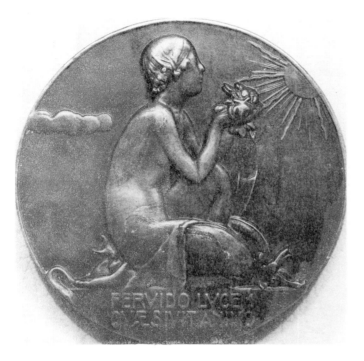

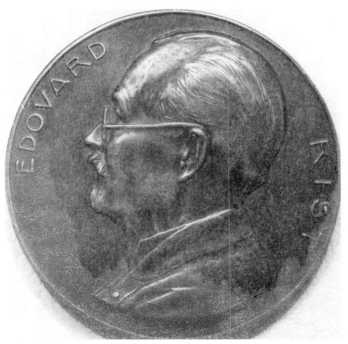

221

Prize medals
awarded by The Royal College
of Physicians of London

William Baly 1814–1861 F. 1846

*By the firm of J. S. and A. B. Wyon, bronze gilt (?) 2 ¼ inches (56 mm.)
diameter*

Obverse. Bust portrait of Baly, head and half shoulders, slightly to left; receding hair; open collar (of gown) *IN HONOREM GULIELMI BALY M.D. OBT. 1861*; signed *J.S.WYON SC.*

Reverse. Round the portico of the building of the College in Pall Mall East lettered *OB PHYSIOLOGIAM FELICITER EXCULTAM*; below *COLL. REG. MED. | LOND.* and *SIR R SMIRKE R.A. ARCHT* and *J.S. & A.B. WYON SC.*

Awarded to *EDGAR ALLEN. 1941* as incised on the rim. The Baly medal was first awarded in 1869.

The College also possesses two bronze strikes.

224   *Ref:* Storer (154); Forrer, VI, pp. 578–79; College *List.*

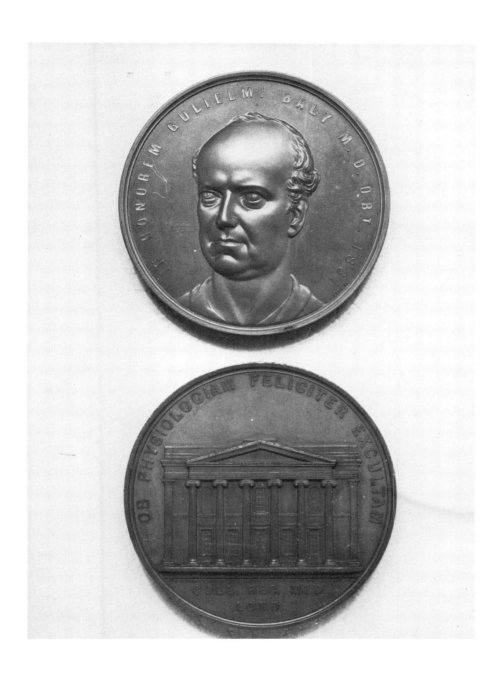

Francis Bisset Hawkins 1796–1895 F. 1826

By Frank Bowcher, silver gilt (?), 3 inches (76 mm.) diameter

Obverse. Head and shoulders portrait of Hawkins, full face; curly hair, full at sides, moustache on upper lip, tuft on lower lip, short beard; he wears coat and waistcoat; lettered *FRANCIS.BISSET HAWKINS.M.D. F.R.C.P.* round upper half, and dated *1796 1895* over shoulders; signed *F.BOWCHER F* on the exergue.

Reverse. Aesculapius, seated receiving Hercules; lettered in upper half *OB SEDVLO | CVLTAM | MEDICINAE CIVILIS | DISCIPLINAM* and signed F.BOWCHER.F on the exergue.

Awarded to Sir George Newman, incised around the edge *SIR GEORGE NEWMAN, G.B.E., K.C.B., 1935.*

The Bisset Hawkins medal was first awarded in 1899.

The College possesses three bronze strikes.

226   *Ref:* Forrer, I, pp. 254–55; Storer (1484); College *List.*

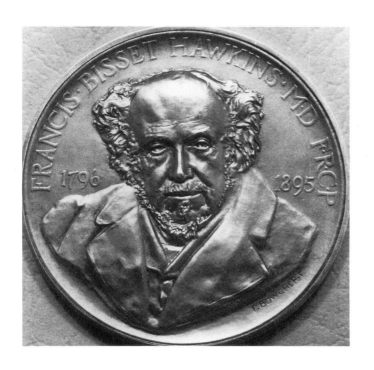

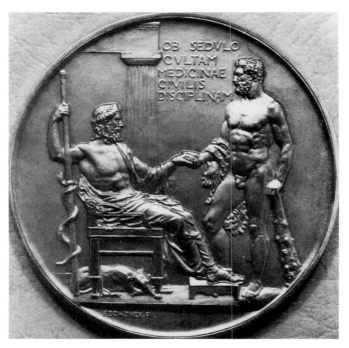

Walter Moxon 1836–1886 F. 1868

By Allan Wyon, gold, 2½ inches (64 mm.) diameter

Obverse. Head and shoulders portrait of Moxon, bearded, looking slightly to right; lettered round it: *IN HONOREM GUALTERI MOXON M.D. MDCCCXXXVI – LXXXVI*; signed *ALLAN WYON SC.*

Reverse. Lettered round an elevation of the fourth building of the College in Pall Mall East: *OB ARTEM MEDICAM STUDIIS ET EXPERIMENTIS AUCTAM*, and, below, *COLL. REG. MED. LOND*, and *SIR R. SMIRKE R.A. ARCHT. ALLAN WYON SC*; on the rim *SIR ARTHUR HURST, M.D., F.R.C.P. 1939.*

The Moxon medal was first awarded in 1891.

Presented by Sir Arthur (Frederick) Hurst, to whom it was awarded.

The College also possesses one bronze strike.

228   *Ref:* Forrer, VI, p. 580; Storer (2504); College *List.*

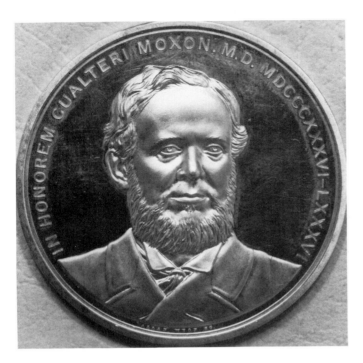

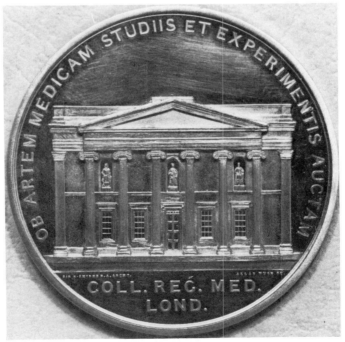

229

Sir Hermann Weber 1823–1918 F. 1859

(Catalogue I, p. 426)

2. By Frank Bowcher, 1894, silver(?), 2 inches (50 mm.) diameter

Obverse. Portrait of Weber in profile to left; head and half shoulders, full hair, side whiskers, beard and moustache; lettered *HERMANN.WEBER.M.D. F.R.C.P. LONDON* round the edge; and dated 1894 on the cutaway.

Reverse. Asklepios seated with Demeter, Apollo and Herakles standing before him (the physician availing himself of the powers of Nature to cure pulmonary tuberculosis); lettered along top edge *WEBER PARKES PRIZE MEDAL* and across bottom *PREVENTION.AND. CVRE | OF.TVBERCVLOSIS.*

The Weber-Parkes medal founded by Weber in 1894 in memory of Dr. Edmund Alexander Parkes 1819–76. The scheme for the reverse is due to Weber himself.

The Weber medal was first awarded in 1897.

Ref: Storer (3747); College *List*; F. P. Weber, *Autobiographical Reminiscences of Sir Hermann Weber*, privately printed, 1919, pl. XIV; *Catalogue* I, 1964, pp. 426–27.

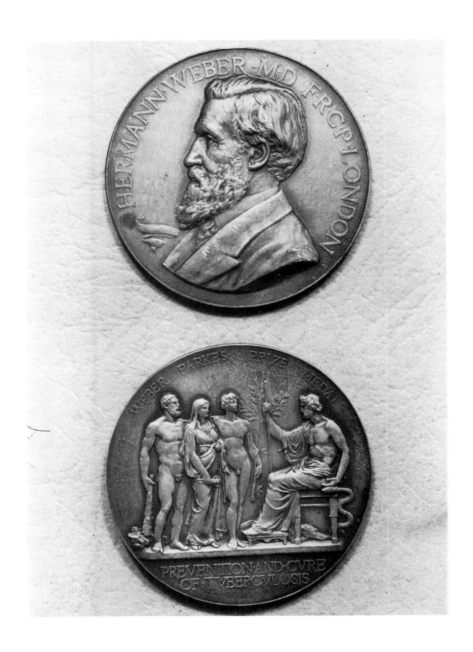

231

Other medals in the possession of the College (not illustrated)

ALBERT, Prince Consort (1819–1861), *see* Queen Victoria.

ALBERT EDWARD, Prince of Wales (1841–1910), *see* King EDWARD VII.

Karl Albert Ludwig ASCHOFF (1866–1942).
By Kraumann.

Sir Benjamin Collins BRODIE (1783–1862).
By William Wyon, 1841.
Struck on his retirement from St. George's Hospital. Award of the Royal College of Surgeons of England.
Storer (483); Freeman (78).

Jean Martin CHARCOT (1825–1893).
By Frédéric de Vernon, 1900.
Struck in honour of Charcot by pupils and admirers on his seventy-fifth birthday. Neurological Conference 1900, awarded to Sir Charles Sherrington, as incised.
Storer (599); Freeman (97) and pl. 21.

Anatole Marie Emile CHAUFFARD (1855–1932).
By G. N. Rispal, 1932 or later.

Jean Baptiste Auguste CHAUVEAU (1827–1917).
By Paul Richer, 1903.
Storer (612); Freeman (100) and pl. 18.

André Victor CORNIL (1837–1917).
By Charles Pillet, 1903.
Storer (688); Freeman (114).

Henri HUCHARD (1844–1910).
By Alfred Boucher, 1903.
In commemoration of twenty-five years of 'médécin des hopitaux'.
Storer (1674); Freeman (249).

King EDWARD VII (1841–1910).
By George T. Morgan, 1873.
International Exhibition of Fine Arts, Industries and Inventions, London, 1873.

GALEN (130–200).
By William Wyon.
The Galen Medal of the Society of Apothecaries.
Forrer, VI, p. 683.

Emile Justin Armand GAUTIER (1837–1920).
By Frédéric de Vernon, 1911.
In honour of fifty years devoted to science.
Storer (1199); Freeman (200) and pl. 21.

Victor GOMOUI (1882–1960).
Roumanian Society of the History of Medicine 1929–1969.

Henri HUCHARD (1844–1910).
By Alfred Boucher, 1903.
In commemoration of twenty-five years as 'médecin des hôpitaux.'
Storer (1674); Freeman (249).

Thomas JEFFERSON (1743–1826).
Jefferson Medical College centenary, Philadelphia, 1925.

Etienne Jules MAREY (1830–1904).
By Paul Richer.
Storer (2364).

Giovanni Battista MORGAGNI (1682–1771).
By Peironi (?)
St. Thomas's Hospital 1899.
Storer (2519).

NAPOLEON Bonaparte.
By Bertrand Andrieu and Julien Marie Jouannin.
Modern strike of medal of 1805.
Ecoles de Medecine.
Storer (6026); Freeman (729).

By Bertrand Andrieu.
La Vaccine 1804.
As described in the note to Freeman (579) with the name of Denon on the reverse.

Pope NICHOLAS V 1398–1455.
University of Glasgow 500th anniversary, 1951.

Louis PASTEUR 1822–1895.
By Louis Oscar Roty.
Two strikes, one in a case lettered *C.S.S. | FRÒM | PASTEUR VALLÈRY-RADOT.*
Centenary of birth, 1922.
Storer (2742); Freeman (394, 395).

Edouard Charles Albert ROBIN (1847–1928).
By Frédéric de Vernon, 1905.
In celebration of his elevation to the rank of commander in the Legion of Honour, and his appointment to the chair of clinical therapy.
Storer (3039); Freeman (455) and pl. 21.

Luigi SACCO (1769–1836).
By Petronio Tadolini, 1802.
Struck by the City of Bologna.
Storer (3104); Freeman (465) and pl. 4.

Johann Ernst Oswald SCHMIEDEBERG (1838–1921).
Storer (3308).

Ignaz Pierre SEMMELWEISS (1818–1865).
By Lajos Béran [c. 1908].
Storer (3338); Freeman (484), a porcelain piece.

Andreas VESALIUS (1514–1564).
By P. Fisch.
Sixth Physiological Congress, Brussels, 1904.
Storer (3619).

Queen VICTORIA (1819–1901).
By Joseph Davis, 1846.
Jugate with Prince Albert.
Brompton Hospital for Consumption, 1844.
Storer (5067); Freeman (614).

By Leonard Charles Wyon, the reverse after a design by Sir John Tenniel.
Seventh International Medical Congress, 1881.
Storer (6307); Freeman (747) and pl. 31.

By George William Desaulles, from two coin portraits by William Wyon and Thomas Brock.
60th Jubilee 1897.
Presented by Dr. S. Monckton Copeman, March 1935.

Rudolph Ludwig Karl VIRCHOW (1821–1902).
By Anton Scharff and Carl Waschmann, 1891.
Replica of gold medallion. Presented on the sitter's seventieth birthday.
Storer (3643); Freeman (536).

Errata Catalogue I

John Arbuthnot 1667–1735 F. 1710 (pp. 28–29)

This portrait has since been found to represent 1st Earl of Mansfield, q.v. (pp. 150–151).

John Elliotson 1791–1868 F. 1822 (pp. 150–151) and Sir Thomas Watson Bt. 1792–1882 F. 1826 P. 1862–1867.

Same portrait reproduced in error on p. 151 and 423. The portrait is of John Elliotson. The correct portrait for Sir Thomas Watson is on p. 425.

Index to Artists